Public Health
in
America

This is a volume in the Arno Press series

PUBLIC HEALTH
IN
AMERICA

See last pages of this volume
for a complete list of titles.

CONSUMPTION IN NEW ENGLAND

and

IS CONSUMPTION CONTAGIOUS?

Henry I[ngersoll] Bowditch

ARNO PRESS

A New York Times Company

New York / 1977

Editorial Supervision: JOSEPH CELLINI

Reprint Edition 1977 by Arno Press Inc.

Consumption in New England is reprinted from a copy in the Columbia University Library.

PUBLIC HEALTH IN AMERICA
ISBN for complete set: 0-405-09804-9
See last pages of this volume for titles.

Manufactured in the United States of America

Publisher's Note: The map facing p.22 has been reproduced in black and white for this edition.

Library of Congress Cataloging in Publication Data

Bowditch, Henry Ingersoll, 1808-1892.
Consumption in New England.

(Public health in America)
Reprint of 2 works, the 1st published in 1862 by Ticknor & Fields, Boston; and the 2d printed in 1864 by D. Clapp, Boston under title: Is consumption ever contagious or communicated by one person to another in any manner?
1. Tuberculosis--New England. 2. Medical geography--New England. 3. Tuberculosis--Etiology. 4. Tuberculosis--Transmission. I. Bowditch, Henry Ingersoll, 1808-1892. Is consumption ever contagious ... 1977. II. Title. III. Title: Is consumption contagious or communicated by one person to another in any manner? IV. Series.
RA644.T7B68 1977 614.5'42'0974 76-25653
ISBN 0-405-09806-5

CONSUMPTION IN NEW ENGLAND:

OR,

LOCALITY ONE OF ITS CHIEF CAUSES.

AN ADDRESS

DELIVERED BEFORE THE

MASSACHUSETTS MEDICAL SOCIETY,

BY HENRY I. BOWDITCH, M.D.

BOSTON:
TICKNOR & FIELDS.
1862.

TO THE

Memory

OF THAT

EXCELLENT MAN AND ACCOMPLISHED PHYSICIAN,

EDWARD AUGUSTUS HOLYOKE,

AND OF HIS

ABLE ASSOCIATES,

THE

FOUNDERS OF THE MASSACHUSETTS MEDICAL SOCIETY;

AND TO MY

LIVING ASSOCIATES,

THE PRESENT FELLOWS OF THE SOCIETY,

TO WHOSE EXTREME COURTESY AND KINDNESS I OWE THE DATA ON WHICH THIS ADDRESS IS FOUNDED,

These Pages

ARE

DEDICATED.

PREFACE.

This pamphlet is an exact transcript of the address I delivered before the Massachusetts Medical Society in May last. The force of facts, presented to me by correspondents, compelled me to resign the commonly received opinion, that consumption is *equally* diffused throughout New England, and to adopt the views of the address, viz.: that there are some spots which have very little of this scourge of the human race, while in other places, and even in particular houses, it prevails to a frightful degree; and moreover, that these spots may be, perhaps, within a very short distance from each other.

Again: facts, as I believe, indicate that dryness of the soil, in the surroundings of any place, is the prominent characteristic of the former, or of places comparatively free from consumption; while dampness of the soil characterizes the latter, or—as they may be aptly called—consumption-breeding districts.

How such effects are produced, I do not and cannot pretend to explain. I am inclined to believe that the explanation will remain long, if not forever, among the *arcana*, of which so many exist in our *apparent* knowledge of the *causes* of disease.

I have delayed publishing until now, because I hoped to have added several letters, &c., confirmatory of the doctrines of the address; but numerous engagements — above all, the absorbing interest that every loyal citizen has in this holy war for National Life and Human Liberty, and my frequent and long absence on professional duties at Washington, in connection with it, and now the commencement of my term of medical instruction at Harvard University — all these have prevented and will prevent me from undertaking, for months to come, any further illustration of the topic of the origin of consumption in New England.

I regret this the less, because—though not as full as could be wished—the address gives the *germ* of the whole idea I would present.

I hopefully commend to the public at large, the perusal of the facts contained in the address; but especially do I present them to the Medical Profession everywhere. I ask practising physicians in New England and elsewhere to examine thoroughly these doctrines and facts by the light of well-recorded statistical data in their own townships, and if they will *prove* me to be in error, I will be the first to acknowledge it.

H. I. B.

BOYLSTON STREET,
Nov. 9, 1862.

TOPOGRAPHICAL DISTRIBUTION

AND

LOCAL ORIGIN

OF

CONSUMPTION IN MASSACHUSETTS.

BY HENRY I. BOWDITCH, M.D.

OF BOSTON.

READ AT THE ANNUAL MEETING OF THE MASS. MED. SOCIETY, MAY 28, 1862.

MR. PRESIDENT AND GENTLEMEN:

AT this dark, but, as I deem it, most glorious epoch in the history of the Republic, and while hosts of armed patriots from all the loyal States are gradually and firmly encircling, as with a wall of fire, the traitors to our country's peace, we—as one small corps of that grand army, whose

"duty is to save"—

have again met, on this our annual festival, for fraternal interchange of thought on topics connected

---

* At an Adjourned Meeting of the Mass. Medical Society, held Oct. 3, 1860, it was

Resolved, "That the Massachusetts Medical Society hereby declares that it does not consider itself as having endorsed or censured the opinions in former published Annual Addresses, nor will it hold itself responsible for any opinions or sentiments advanced in any future similar addresses."

Resolved, "That the Committee on Publication be directed to print a statement to that effect at the commencement of each Annual Address which may hereafter be published."

with the science or art of our noble, but peaceful profession. The heart of the Nation is in mourning for her soldiers slain in the beauty of their young lives and of their heroic deeds, on the battle-fields of our common country. We, too, lament the loss of many of our well-known and respected fellow soldiers in the battle of life, who, since our last gathering, have left our ranks only to join the mightier hosts of the dead. A few moments spent in commemoration of their virtues will tend to hallow this hour, which, year after year, we devote to professional discourse.

Not less than twenty-seven of our number have died during the past year ; a larger number than has ever been known before within the same period of time. Most of them filled, to the entire satisfaction of the various communities in which they lived, the sacred office of Family Physician. They need no higher or sweeter eulogium ; for that office, worthily filled, carries within itself as rare a combination of virtues possessed and of duties done as usually falls to the lot of man.

I shall not, I hope, be deemed unjust to the memory of others, or as using the language of unmeaning panegyric, if I allude more distinctly and personally to two of them ; one of whom was but recently our President, while the place of the other as Secretary has become vacant only within the last few weeks. As officers of this Association, therefore, if for no other reason, we owe to their memories, at the present hour, our tribute of respect.

Dr. LUTHER V. BELL* was a member of a family in New Hampshire, illustrious for its talents and for the high positions held by it in the service of the State. After a brief career as a practitioner of medicine in his native State, he was called, as almost the immediate successor of the late excellent Dr. Wyman, to the charge of the Asylum for the Insane at Somerville. During the twenty years that Dr. Bell was there, the institution sustained its previously high repute. His serene deportment, his pure life, his sagacity, his unswerving integrity, and his many professional accomplishments, commanded the respect of all connected with the Asylum and of the community at large. His Annual Reports were eagerly sought after, and were remarkable for their clear good sense. Although one or more times, in consequence of ill-health, he resigned, he was persuaded to remain at his post for a certain time longer. It was hard to fill his place. After he left the Asylum, in 1856, he spent his hours in dignified retirement in the bosom of his family, only occasionally emerging therefrom to mingle as leader in political life, or to attend in consultation on cases related to his own specialty. In the Courts of Law of Massachusetts, his opinion on medico-legal questions of insanity was highly prized.

While thus resting from his labors, came "this glorious uprising of a great people," and the North as one man sprung to arms, at the fall of Sumter. Dr. Bell felt that the hour had come for every man

---

* Appendix A—Memorial.

to do his whole duty. He applied for and immediately received the appointment of Surgeon to the 11th Regiment, Massachusetts Volunteers. Contrary to the wishes of many, and the advice of others, who thought his health too feeble to endure the fatigues of camp life, he promptly obeyed the orders that summoned him to the banks of the Potomac. His talents and worth soon raised him to the rank of Brigade Surgeon. Soon after he left, a letter was sent to him by a friend, expressive of high admiration of the step Dr. Bell had taken, and wishing him a friendly "God speed." Two manly responses were subsequently received from him, from which I have been allowed to quote certain passages, showing some of his views of the present crisis and his self-sacrificing patriotism.

Under date of Sept. 13th, 1861, after alluding to the opposition of friends to his assuming, in his feeble health, the rough duties of the camp, and of the suggestion of others that when his "enthusiasm had collapsed" he "would pine for the quiet of his amply-provided home," he remarks, "I never for a moment gave heed to those who prophesied a disposition to draw back. Because, never experiencing any other enthusiasm beyond a strong impulse of duty, I knew their premises were ill-founded."

Again, after stating the numerous difficulties he had had to contend with, "yet," adds he, "with all these drawbacks I have never had a sick day, or a sad hour, independently of what a father must feel at the thought of four motherless children away from him; nor has the thought ever crossed my mind of leaving the service until the last blow is struck upon the life of this atrocious rebellion."

On another occasion, alluding to the objections — risk to life, family ties, &c. — urged by some against the entrance of a young man into the army at the present time, he says, "At all events, we have only one life. What better use of it than to give it to the holy cause of our country? Had my eldest son, who died during his first year of college life, been spared, I would cheerfully have consented to his bearing arms in this hour of emergency."

How fitting it seems that such words of loftiest patriotism should have been sealed only a few months afterwards by his own death, while in the service of his then humiliated country, but now on the very verge of triumph!

Dr. Bell was seized with an acute thoracic attack, following what was supposed to be rheumatism. His dyspnœa was intense for a short time; but, as we learn from his attendants, his confidence never forsook him. He knew that his last illness was reached. Though his sufferings at times were great, he conversed freely with the Chaplain upon high religious topics; and, commending himself to God, quietly expired under the ample folds of his dear country's flag. I quote only the language of one who knew whereof he spoke, when I add that, in the death of our beloved friend and learned associate, the officers of the staff, from the highest to the lowest, felt that their "light" had been extinguished. Stronger, more intellectual, perhaps physically braver men there might be; and the loss of each other one could be readily supplied by an associate equally worthy. But into the magic circle of good and winning qualities possessed by Dr. Bell, and which made him thus the electric light of the staff, none else could enter. Let us all thank God for this bright, this beautiful Ideal, which death has now made of our associate's noble life—sanctified, too, as it was, by a patriot's death.

Our excellent friend and valued Secretary, Dr. J. B. ALLEY,* passed years of the most patient suffering from hereditary phthisis, to the progress of which he ever looked forward, with the most open-eyed cheerfulness, in certain anticipation of his future fate. Unremitting in his quiet but efficient, pious, toil for the good of others, eminently faithful and reliable in the performance of every duty, he was a truly Christian Gentleman, in the broadest signification of that term. I could not find it in my heart to say less of him. I need say no more.

In taking, Gentlemen, a subject for my address on this occasion, I shall follow out the idea quaintly suggested by that admirable man and sweet English writer, George Herbert, when describing what the country parson's sermon should be. "The world," he remarks, "is full of these composures, yet every man's own is fittest, readiest and most savory to him." Some of you have already listened to my previous, imperfect discussions on the topic I shall present, for I have twice before at our annual meetings, at

* Appendix—Memorial.

Springfield in 1855, and again at Boston in 1856, made brief allusions to an investigation I was at that time carrying on, as a Committee of this Society — namely:

On the Topographical Distribution and Local Origin of Consumption in Massachusetts.

Since that time, my attention has been constantly directed to this important subject. My convictions have become more and more settled upon the essential truthfulness of the views I, in 1855 and '56, only tremblingly enunciated. I have obtained since then, through private investigations and from various correspondents, not only in Massachusetts, but in New England, still more ample proof. My own daily practice in connection with this terrible scourge, said by Keith Johnston* to be endemic, par excellence, in New England, is perpetually modified by my stern belief in principles then stated imperfectly. I should therefore consider myself really culpable were I to waste your valuable time in any abstruse and polemical questions on therapeutics, or the general practice of medicine, and should neglect to speak on that subject, which, for eight years past, has engrossed so much of my thoughts.

The facts I shall lay before you, and the principles I believe fairly deducible therefrom, involve the

---

* Geographical Distribution of Health and Disease, by W. Keith Johnston. Edinburgh, 1854.

Dr. Josiah Curtis (Mass. State Registration, 1859, page 71) virtually agrees to this when he says that three die of consumption in New England for every two persons in Great Britain of the same disease.

question of the proof or otherwise of the existence of a Great Primal Law in the Development of Consumption in Massachusetts, and probably New England, and possibly of a still wider scope, *not hitherto distinctly recognized.* Attention to this law by our ancestors, and by ourselves at the present hour, would, as I believe, have saved, and would still be saving, hecatombs of human beings that are now annually sacrificed. Holding most firmly to this opinion, you will readily understand my eager anxiety to convince not only you, my associates and efficient collaborators in this investigation, but, through you, the whole community, of its vital importance to the present and still more to future generations in New England, and possibly other parts of our country.

But in addition to the intrinsic worth of the subject to be discussed, I claim your candid, and, if possible, close attention to the remarks I shall make, for another reason, viz.: The inferences I shall make, and the Law of Consumption Development I shall try to support, are merely the summing up of data furnished to me by yourselves. I stand, therefore, now before you the exponent of your own (unconscious, perhaps, it may be on the part of many of you) medical opinion. For you are all aware that to the courtesy and to that fine *esprit de corps* I have always found in the Massachusetts Medical Society, spread as it is over all the Old Bay State, from beyond the Berkshire Hills to the Atlantic Coast, I owe *all* the chief facts and statements upon which this opinion is founded.

The two following propositions contain the essential points of this address :—

First. A residence on or near a damp soil, whether that dampness be inherent in the soil itself, or caused by percolation from adjacent ponds, rivers, meadows, marshes or springy soils, is one of the primal causes of consumption in Massachusetts, probably in New England, and possibly in other portions of the globe.

Second. Consumption can be checked in its career, and possibly, nay probably, prevented in some instances, by attention to this law.

The essential truths thus enunciated I am ready to defend against all mere assertions of individual opinion, however much those assertions may appear to sustain the reverse of these propositions. I pray you not to judge hastily, but if any remarks I make seem not warranted by the present state of medical knowledge, suspend awhile your judgments, and look not only at *my* facts, but open your own eyes and your intellects to a fair and thorough examination of similar facts, that may be really occurring within the rounds of *your* daily professional life. If you do this, it may happen, as it has happened to myself, and also to one who was, at first, a very decided opponent, an aged and very excellent practitioner in New Hamphsire. We both became convinced, in spite of our own preconceived notions, solely by the evidence of actual phenomena, occurring, as it were, under our very eyes.

I lay down now before you, as among my *Medical Axioms*, the following statements:—

1st. *Consumption is not, as some writers have contended, endemic equally in every part of New England;* but there are some localities where it is very rife, and others where it is vastly less destructive than in the State at large.

2d. *There is a law*, hitherto scarcely noticed, or but vaguely hinted at by one or two individual writers, but (as I believe) *never proved* until now, *which is one of the main causes, if not the sole cause, of this unequal topographical distribution of consumption in New England.*

3d. *This law is intimately connected with, and apparently dependent on, the humidity of the soils, on or near which stand the towns, villages, or even single houses, where consumption prevails.*

4th. *The existence of this law of soil-moisture, as one of the prime causes of consumption in New England*, can be proved, as I think, by several lines of argument, resting on actual facts obtained either from public or private records, statistical data, or the opinions of physicians, practising medicine in various parts of New England.

These lines of proof, or of argument, are drawn from the following sources:—

I. Massachusetts State Registration Reports.

II. Medical Opinion of Massachusetts, as embodied in the returns made to me, as a Committee of this Society — these returns consisting of written reports from resident physicians of one hundred and eighty-three towns.

III. Actual Statistics of deaths by consumption, received from such correspondents. Some of these statistics are but *incidentally* mentioned, while others are from towns, districted and carefully examined with reference to the relative prevalence of consumption in the different districts. In some of the most important of these, the examination was made without my correspondent or myself being aware of the existence of any law such as that which I shall present at this time.

IV. Peculiarities of certain towns and of villages in the same townships, in some of which consumption is quite prevalent, and in others much less so; these differences being connected most closely with corresponding differences in the amount of moisture of the soil of said places.

V. Certain well-known houses, which, in various towns, are known by the inhabitants and physicians to have been long noted as the abode of consumption, and in some of which several families have been, during the past fifty years, cut off by the disease, without the least suspicion, on the part of the occupants, of the fatal position in which the houses were placed.

VI. Confirmatory facts, statistics and opinions from Rhode Island, Maine and New Hampshire.

VII. The medical statistics given in the Report on the health of the United States Army, strongly supporting the idea of the existence of the same law, and the operation of it over the whole of the United States.

VIII. Results of my own practice since I first became convinced of the truth of the law—said results consisting of *(a)* Statistics from my private medical records; *(b)* Results actually derived from my choice of localities for consumptive patients, based on a belief in the law.

IX. Apparent exceptions to the law.

It will, of course, be impossible to do anything more than briefly allude to each of these various lines of proof; and while doing so, I must ask you to believe in the truthfulness of what I quote from the voluminous manuscript reports and letters, received chiefly from yourselves and from some excellent and zealous physicians in Maine, New Hampshire and Rhode Island.

These reports and these letters should be kept among other valuable manuscripts of the Society. They embody not only the present medical opinion about consumption and its causes, in Massachusetts, but much incidental matter of importance to Public Hygiene. I hope, at some future time, the Society will have portions of them published.

I. State Registration Reports.

The following table is mainly founded on statistics of four years, or between 1849 and 1852, inclusive. The last column, containing the proportion of deaths by consumption to the population, includes five years, viz., 1849–'53 inclusive.*

* State Registration, Report 11th, pages 70–136, and Report 12th, p. 162.

TABLE I.

*Showing Consumption slightly more prevalent in the Atlantic than in the Inland Counties.**

INLAND COUNTIES.	Deaths by Consumption, 1849 to 1852.	Deaths by all Diseases, 1849 to 1852.	Per centages of Deaths by Consumption to all Deaths.	One Person dies by Consumption in every †	ATLANTIC COUNTIES.	Deaths by Consumption, 1849 to 1852.	Deaths by all Diseases, 1849 to 1852.	Per centages of Deaths by Consumption to all Deaths.	One Person dies by Consumption in every †
Berkshire......	591	2783	21.27	67 per.	Barnstable...	473	1869	25.30	60 per.
Franklin.......	419	1733	24.17	56 "	Bristol.......	1172	4920	23.82	50 "
Hampden......	720	3529	20.40	55 "	Dukes.....} Nantucket..}	214	738	28.99	50 "
Hampshire....	520	2355	22.08	53 "					
Middlesex......	2292	10802	21.21	53 "	Plymouth...	894	3223	27.73	47 "
Norfolk........	1046	5168	20.22	58 "	Essex........	2153	9369	22.97	48 "
Worcester......	2080	9287	22.39	48 "	Suffolk.......	2696	16934	15.91	42 "

* 22.44 of all deaths in Massachusetts are caused by consumption. Vide Reg. Rep. 1853; also 1859, p. 71.
† Data for 5 years, 1849 to 1853. (See Appendix.)

Middlesex and Norfolk Counties are placed among the inland counties, while they do, in reality, touch the Atlantic coast. Strictly speaking, Middlesex does not touch the *coast*, though one small point projects down *near* it. In Norfolk, I have considered that the vast proportion of all the inhabitants of the county are subjected to inland influences. All the table is intended to prove, is, that apparently even the imperfect State Registration indicates that consumption is not equally prevalent in all parts of the Commonwealth; and second, that probably it prevails a little more on the coast, or where coast influences are exerted on the inhabitants, than it does where the inland influences prevail.

Again, it will be remarked that Berkshire, the most western county, about 200 miles from the Atlantic, hilly, with warm valleys, seems less afflicted than any in the State.

Worcester shows apparently the influence of its large central city—"the heart of the Commonwealth"—in the frequency of consumption.

Similar remarks may be made of Suffolk, of which Boston is almost the sole influencing power. Barnstable, on the contrary, on the coast, and doubly exposed to coast influences, has two advantages over its companions. It is a long, comparatively narrow peninsula, and composed almost entirely of a sandy porous soil. Of the advantage derived from these two circumstances, we shall have hereafter opportunities of being convinced, as we proceed in our investigations.

II.—Medical Opinion on the Prevalence of Consumption in Massachusetts.

This opinion is based upon answers made by resident Physicians of one hundred and eighty-three, out of the three hundred and twenty-five townships in Massachusetts. The answers were replies to the two following questions:—

1st, Is any portion of your town peculiarly liable to the prevalence of consumption?

2d, If so, what, if any, are the peculiarities of the spot?

These questions were introduced into a list I had previously prepared of fifteen other questions—the answers to which would enable a reader to judge of the hygienic condition of the township, or localities in it, and obtain some idea of the social and industrial state of the inhabitants.*

* For questions and names of Correspondents, see App. B.

I had hoped to compare these returns with the State Registration Reports of Deaths and Diseases. This was impossible, owing to the imperfect returns made by State officials. I introduced the two questions, above given, rather unwillingly, because I had no belief that any good would result, feeling confident, as I suppose the majority of you are, that consumption prevails equally over every portion of New England. I yielded, however, to the suggestion, because of the sagacity of him who made it.

By dint of repeated circulars, during a period of nearly three years, I obtained returns from all the towns of the Commonwealth. Of the one hundred and eighty-three physicians, I have no reason to believe that a single one held the opinion that I must enunciate, or fail to express what really their data compel me to say. I mention this, in order that you may understand, still more distinctly, how little I, and I think others who now agree with me, have been guided by preconceived notions on the subject. Still further, two of my correspondents evidently recognized the existence of *some unknown* law of development of consumption. They had, in fact, by their own careful investigations, elaborated the influence of the very law, I shall bring forward, and one wrote to me upon the existence of some unknown law; but he could not generalize enough from the imperfect data of one town, even to get a glimpse of what soon became clear to me, who was able to collate returns from all quarters of the State.

Before giving the *resumé* of these returns, and from which I infer the "*Medical Opinion*" of the State, let me meet an objection urged, at first, by some of the ablest of the profession, and by others, against the value of "medical opinion." "In these days of skepticism, who believes in anything dependent on mere medical opinion?" Such was really the objection instantly raised by one, who formerly was an able opponent. I recognize and acknowledge, to a certain degree, at least, the justice of the palpable sneer against the slight grounds on which medical opinion is but too often based. But I totally deny its applicability to the present case, and for the following reason. In the answers to the two questions above named, there is not involved the consideration of any abstruse question in medicine, but simply the statement of the existence or non-existence of facts, viz., the more frequent occurrence or non-occurrence of consumption in certain localities, and a specification of the peculiarities, if any, of these localities. For aught I can see, we may believe a physician's report of such facts, as much as we would believe the statement made by any intelligent witness of a certain fact. I not only claim this, but I assert that we ought to take the statements made by physicians, educated men, as those made by a class of persons, far above the average of witnesses on any subject. Now this Medical Opinion, which I shall present to you, is simply my inference from statements made to me by physicians, who have had no concert with one another, and must have been without the least suspicion of what I may have thought, or may have been supposed to wish them to say upon the subject. These facts have occurred in their own townships, while engaged in their daily routines of medical practice. I have simply laid out before me their returns, and from such data have elaborated the following classification of the towns of the Commonwealth. Logically, I think I can claim any inference, that can be justly drawn therefrom, as the *real* medical opinion of the State, even if each and every one of my correspondents, looking at the subject from his own stand-point, may, at first sight, be disposed to deny that he admits the truth of such inference.

All the answers to the circulars, have come from physicians, except in three instances, where there were no physicians in the towns; and in these cases, intelligent citizens have replied.

Two hundred and twelve have answered more or less elaborately, the two questions above stated, viz., by one hundred and eighty-three were given medical opinions, and, at times, statistics *incidentally;* by ten, valuable statistical data were procured for the special elucidation of the subject; by nineteen, either doubtful or opposing statements to the views, entertained in this address, were given; by twenty-one, miscellaneous statements were made on the hygienic condition of the towns, but not bearing at all upon the topics herein discussed.

Finally, from the remainder, a little more than one third of the towns in the State, I have had simply monosyllabic, negative, answers to the two special questions, and equally monosyllabic, but definite, returns to all other questions. These returns cannot, of course, be used in this discussion, save so far as this, viz., that a certain number of physicians of the Commonwealth have not observed any peculiarities in the prevalence of consumption, in different portions of their towns. The fact, however, that a phenomenon, not very palpable even to the most acute observer, is not seen by every one, is no proof of the non-existence of that phenomenon, especially when it is in agreement with the elaborate, well-gathered statistical data of a certain number.

Climometrician

Rush 66
Bowditch 92

The one hundred and eighty-three townships above-named may be classified as follows:—

First, Townships in which, according to the opinion of resident Physicians, consumption is *quite rife.* (Colored *red* on map*)	28
Second, Those in which resident Physicians find *certain localities* unusually subject to consumption, and more so than are the towns generally. (Colored with *red line* around township)	54
Third, Those combining both of these qualities, viz., townships in which the disease is *quite common* in every part, and still more so in certain localities. (Colored with *a red cross*)	21
Fourth, Those in which it is more rarely seen in the town as a whole, but in which are found certain localities *peculiarly afflicted* by it. (Colored *blue,* with *red lines around*)	23
Fifth, Those in which consumption is rare. (Colored *blue*)	57
Total,	183

In order to give at a glance the whole results, I submit the following table, compiled from these returns.

---

* See Map.

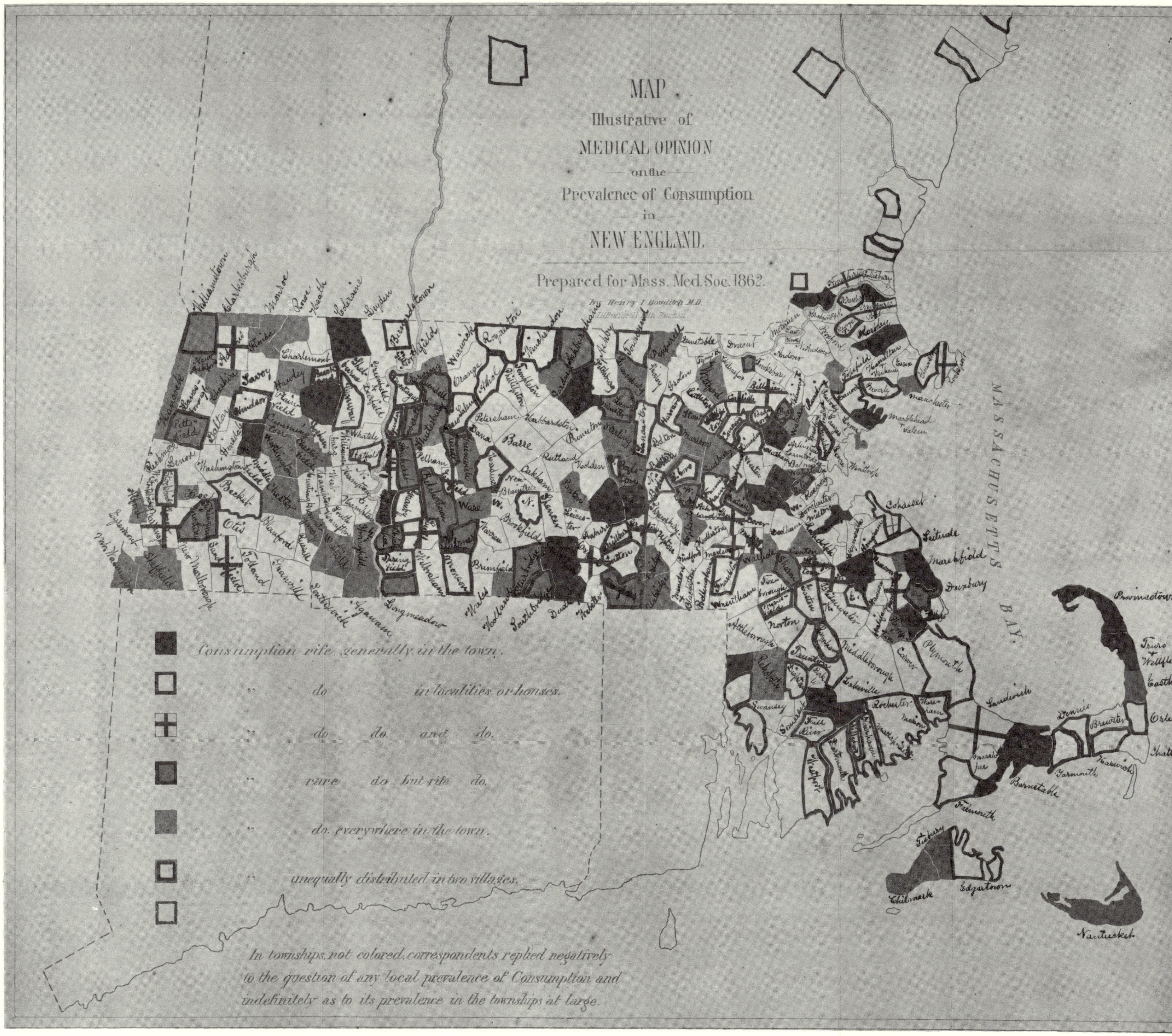
MAP
Illustrative of
MEDICAL OPINION
on the
Prevalence of Consumption
in
NEW ENGLAND.
Prepared for Mass. Med. Soc. 1862.
by Henry I. Bowditch M.D.
J.H.Bufford's Lith. Boston.
MASSACHUSETTS BAY.
Consumption rife generally in the town.
" do in localities or houses.
" do do. and do.
" rare do but rife do.
" do. everywhere in the town.
" unequally distributed in two villages.
In townships, not colored, correspondents replied negatively to the question of any local prevalence of Consumption and indefinitely as to its prevalence in the townships at large.

TABLE II.

Showing the opinions of Resident Physicians in 183 Towns on the Prevalence of Consumption in the Townships or parts of them, and a comparison of this Prevalence with the amount of Moisture and Dryness of the Townships or Localities.

No. of Towns from which data are obtained.	Consumption prevails.	Dryness a prominent characteristic (i. e. "towns are exposed," "dry, mountainous," "sheltered," "dry," "island," "peninsula.")*	Per centages. — DRY or INSULAR.	Moisture a prominent characteristic (i.e. "exposed moist," "on the shore," "near river," "pond," "meadow," "springy soil," "foggy.")	Per centages. — MOIST.	OTHER INFLUENCES. Bad Habits.	Factory.	Hereditary.	Bleak Exposure.	Valley, Medium.	Doubtful.
28	Generally.	In 6 Towns.	21.42	In 20 Towns.	71.42						2
54	In certain localities	In none.	......	In 50 localities.	92.59	2	1		1		
21	Generally and in certain localities.	In 6.	28.57	In 14 Towns.	66.66						1
		In none.	......	In 16 localities.	76.19		1		2		2
23	Rarely, but much in certain localities.	In 13.	56.52	In 6 Towns.	26.08				2	1	1
		In none.	......	In 13 localities.	56.52		5	1		2	2
57	Rarely.	In 37.	64.91	In 9 Towns.	15.78						11
183		62	Average, 24.48 are dry.	128	Av. 57.87 are moist.						

* For reasons why "islands and peninsulas" are here included, see remarks in this Address on the subject of "Places of residence favorable for Consumptives."

This table may be thus read:—Of those townships where consumption is, in the opinion of resident physicians, *rife*, nearly three quarters (71.42 per ct.) are *damp*; whereas in other townships, where the disease is on the same authority said to be of rare occurrence, *dryness* is the characteristic, in nearly the same proportion (viz., 64.91 per ct.). This becomes still more manifest, if we examine the other data in the table. For example, we find 92.59 per cent. of all those parts of 54 townships which are, for some heretofore, unknown reason, more subject than others to the prevalence of consumption, are moist, and *not one is described as dry!*

Again, of the 21 townships said to have rather more of the disease than other towns have of it, 66.66 per cent. of them are moist. These townships have localities, in which consumption prevails inordinately. Now, in these localities, the per centages in regard to moisture are vastly augmented, 76.19 of them being moist, and *none being described as dry.*

Finally, of 23 townships, in which consumption is thought to be *rarely* prevalent, we find 56.52 per cent. are dry; 26.08 moist; but in these same townships there are localities, peculiarly subject to the disease, and here we find the result similar to that given above, viz., 56.52 of these localities are moist, and *none are dry.*

We thus see, first, that, in the five classes of townships reported upon, dampness of the soil seems to prevail as the prominent characteristic of the *townships*, in which consumption prevails; and second, this becomes much more evident in the smaller localities and parts of towns where consumption is rife, in *not a single one of which is dryness noticed!* but, on the contrary, very large per centages (92, 76, and 56) are wet. I think you must agree with me that the following proposition seems fairly deducible from the statements given:—

Medical opinion in Massachusetts, as deduced from the written statements of resident physicians in 183 *towns, tends strongly to prove, though perhaps not affording perfect proof of, the existence of a law in the development of consumption in Massachusetts, which law has for its central idea, that dampness of the soil of any township or locality is intimately connected, and probably as cause and effect, with the prevalence of consumption in that township or locality.*

III.—Actual Statistics of deaths by Consumption received from my Correspondents.

This species of proof is, of course, the most valuable, but, at the same time, very difficult to procure. For several years, I have endeavored to persuade some of my correspondents to classify different districts of their several towns, according to the characteristics of the soil or amount of water in these portions, and also to procure the exact number of deaths by consumption and by all diseases, in the same districts, and, if possible, the number of inhabitants of each. To obtain such data, one must have not only very obliging correspondents, but likewise persons of some leisure, and, still more, men imbued with a real love for scientific investigations into the mysteries of medical topography and vital statistics. A few such it has been my good fortune to have had. And although their statistics are few, they are of such a nature as not only to support the results obtained from medical opinion, but seemed to give more definiteness of outline, to what may perhaps be a law of dampness of the soil, as a cause of consumption, already foreshadowed by medical opinion.

The statistics are of two kinds:—

1st, Those incidentally and cursorily given by correspondents in connection with their general accounts of the hygienic condition of various towns.

2d, Statistics of deaths by consumption and by all diseases, or population, procured from the various districts in the townships. This second series is vastly the more valuable one of the two; and it is evident that any such data, if procured from a perfectly unbiassed source, and if confirmatory of medical opinion and of less elaborate statistics, become of great value, although they may be few in number.

I present the following Table (III.), as showing the first kind of statistics. It may be called the *Table of Incidental Statistics*, to distinguish it from that which I would call *Table of Elaborate Statistics*, to be given subsequently.

We may read this table as follows:—Column first says that in two thirds (8-12) of the twelve towns in which consumption prevails generally, moisture of the places is a prominent feature; while *only one sixth* (2-12) *are dry.* Column second indicates that of nine particular localities where consumption prevails, eight ninths (8-9) are moist or are near moist places, one has a variable state, and *none are dry.*

TABLE III.

Made by comparing the Statistics of Deaths by Consumption, as given incidentally *by my Correspondents in various Towns and localities in Massachusetts, with the hygienic condition (chiefly in regard to the amount of moisture of the soil) of said Townships and Localities, as given by the same Correspondents.*

Characteristics of the Town or Locality.	CONSUMPTION PREVAILS IN TOWN OR LOCALITY						
	Generally.	Locally.	Generally and Locally.		Rarely.	Rarely in Town, but much locally.	
			Gen.	*Loc.*		*Gen.*	*Loc.*
Dryness..........	2 towns.	....	2 towns.	....	12 towns.	6 towns.	....
Moisture	8 "	6 towns.	10 "	11 towns	1 "	1 "	4 towns.
Moisture near	....	2 "	....	....	....	....	1 "
Sheltered, warm ..	....	....	....	....	1 "	....	....
Diluvial, Sand near	....	....	....	....	1 "	....	....
Low	....	....	....	....	....	....	1 "
Variable Climate..	....	1 "	2 "	....	1 "	....	....
Promontory	....	....	...	....	2 "	....	....
Exp. to N. Winds.	....	....	....	....	....	....	1 "
do. not changeable	....	....	....	....	....	1 "	....
High	....	....	....	....	....	1 "	....
Medium	....	....	....	....	1 "	....	....
Doubtful	2 "	....	....	1 "	....	....	....
Totals.	12	9	14	12	19	9	7

Columns third and fourth show that of fourteen townships where consumption prevails generally, and also locally, in an especial manner, five sevenths (5-7) of the townships are moist, one seventh (1-7) variable, one seventh (1-7) is dry; while of the consumption-bearing localities, eleven twelfths (11-12) are damp, and one twelfth (1-12) is doubtful — *not one is dry.*

Column fifth declares that of nineteen towns, that

have less consumption than others, twelve (12-19) *are dry*, only one (1-19) is moist. The others have influences, either insular, or medium, or tending to dryness. In other words, where consumption is less prevalent, there less moisture is found in townships or localities.

Columns sixth and seventh illustrate in one town the results produced in columns five and two; two thirds of the townships where consumption is rare, being *dry*, while localities in the same townships, known to have an undue amount of consumption, are more than half of them moist, or "near moist," "low," or "exposed" places.

I am permitted therefore, I think, to assert, that:

Statistics gathered incidentally from my Correspondents sustain, as far as they sustain any opinion, on the question before us, the views we have drawn from Medical Opinion.

But I shall now present statistical evidence, which not only sustains the results of medical opinion and incidental statistics, but seems to *present strong presumptive evidence* that there is a certain, almost fixed ratio in the prevalence of consumption, according to the amount of dampness in the particular location.

In order to present this part of my subject more clearly, I have prepared the following table from data obtained at my special request. In it are found, I think, accurate mortuary statistics. Though few in number, a careful survey of their bearings upon the question seems to sustain all preceding statements, and suggests further and more exact ideas of the influence of the law. The following inferences are fairly deducible from the table (IV.):

1st. Six (Acton, Cohasset, Townsend, Granby, Northboro', West Newbury) out of eight towns, carefully districted with reference to locality, afford mortuary statistics each sustaining, more or less fully, all my previous assertions and inferences. One (Boston) affords doubtful results, the statistics of the native population being in accordance with previous results, while the Irish seem to have had a greater proportion of deaths on the hill than in the lower, and apparently, more damp locality. Both of these localities, however, are equal in filth and in all the concomitants of an over-crowded Irish population. Finally, one (Royalston) is reported to have had over five per cent. more of deaths from consumption in the dry than in the wet localities. I do not pretend to account for this, but would simply draw attention to the fact of the enormous per centages of consumption, compared to total deaths in both parts of the town (32.51 and 38.22), indicating certainly a very peculiar township. I know nothing of its peculiarities, and I cannot suggest any explanation of the apparent anomaly. With these exceptions, we may say that from four to fifty per cent. more of consumption deaths are found in the wet than in the dry localities of the townships.

2d. Some of the towns present, in their data, a *more or less regular gradation in the prevalence of consumption, according to the amount of moisture in or near the various localities.*

TABLE IV.

Names of Towns.	Data on which the Table rests.	Number of Deaths by Consumption. In Dry Localities. All Deaths.	Consump.	Per cent. to total deaths.	Localities of Medium Moist. All Deaths.	Consump.	Per cent. to total deaths.	Clayey Subsoil. All Deaths.	Consump.	Per cent. to total deaths.	Localities near Dampness. All Deaths.	Consump.	Per cent. to total deaths.	Low, damp Localities. All Deaths.	Consump.	Per cent. to total deaths.
Acton	305 deaths. 45 by consumption, fr. 1846 to 1856, inclusive.	180	9	5.00	....		......	....		......	....		......	125	33	26.40
Cohasset	433 deaths, 81 by consumption, fr. 1844 to 1857.	59	9	15.25	102	19	18.62	....		......	192	53	27.60	....		......
Boston (1 yr.)*, 1856	Amr. 87 deaths. 21 Consum.	53	11	20.75										34	10	29.41
	Irish. 202 deaths. 45 Cons.	44	11	25.00	....		......	....		......	....		......	158	34	21.51
Royalston	Pop. 1469.† 198 deaths, 68 by Con. fr. 1851 to '59 inclusive.	34	13	38.23										163	53	32.51

NORTHBORO'............	Pop. 1568. 13 yrs.	One dies by Consumption in every 74.5 persons.	One dies by Consumption in every 29.7 persons.	....	......	....	......	One dies by Consumption in every 23.69 persons.
W. NEWBURY ‡..........	Pop. 1746. 213 deaths, 43 by Con. fr. May 1, '44 to Ap. 30, '54. 10 yrs.	One dies by Consumption in every 76.55 inhabitants.	One dies by Consumption in every 52.06 inhabitants.					One dies by Consumption in every 24.95 inhabitants.
		Per cent. to estimated Pop.	*Per cent. to estimated Pop.*		*Per cent. to estimated Pop.*			*Per cent to estimated Pop.*
TOWNSEND §............	43 by consumption, fr. 1848 to 1853, inclusive.	16.36	19.11		25.85			30.85

* These statistics were procured from the City Registrar. They are from four districts in the City, viz.: two elevated, Beacon and Fort Hills, and two lower and damper districts, Harrison Avenue and South Cove. Beacon Hill and Harrison Avenue districts are occupied by Americans; the other two by Irish.

† In "dry locality," Royalston, population 350; in "low, damp" locality, 1100.

‡ The returns from West Newbury become more distinct and peculiarly instructive as to the (apparent, at least) influence of moisture, as productive of Consumption, if we classify the districts into northern and southern, or those "adjacent to the river," with "clayey subsoil" drying slowly in the spring, and those separated from the river by a range of hills, and having much less clayey subsoil, being thereby warmer and drier. Thus:—

In districts No. 1, 2, 3 (Map), northern or river districts, one dies by consumption in every 36.31.
In districts No. 4, 5, 6 (Map), southern, and drier, warmer, one dies by consumption in every 59.37.

§ These statistics of Townsend show the relative proportion of deaths in the different districts, according to the population in each, as deduced from the absolute number of scholars in each district. To those unacquainted with Massachusetts, and consequently unaware of the almost universal education of children in the country towns of the State, this method of arriving at the relative population may seem very indefinite. I certainly should have preferred more exact returns; but it is evident my correspondent could not, without taking a census of each district, have obtained any returns more accurate than this approximation to the exact truth, obtained from the records of the district schools.

TABLE IV.—*(Continued).* GRANBY, *May* 1, 1843, *to Dec.* 1, 1855.

Returns.	Population.	Deaths. All Deaths.	Deaths. Consumption	Per cent. of Deaths by Consumpt'n to total Deaths.	Per cent. of Deaths by Consumpt'n to Pop.
Physician's Returns.					
Moist Districts........	375	....	29	....	7.73
Remainder of Town....	625	....	12	....	1 92
Town Clerk's Returns.					
Moist Districts........	....	81	36*	44.44	....
Remainder of Town....	....	102	17	16.66	....

* The discrepancy between the returns of Physician and Town Clerk, is owing to the Clerk having probably recorded some cases as consumption, which merely *appeared* to be such.

In one of them (Townsend), this fact is most extraordinarily well marked. Before receiving these data, I had become convinced that dampness of the soil did have an important influence on the prevalence of consumption, over large tracts of country. But these returns from Townsend indicated that there was, perhaps, a law of consumptive development, that would show itself within much narrower limits. It definitely foreshadowed differences in the deaths by consumption, in spots of the same townships, *very near—almost contiguous to each other*, but which presented very different geological characteristics. Such being the fact, and these data having had such an important influence over my own mind, in its views of this whole subject, I may perhaps be pardoned for alluding still more particularly to them. My correspondent entered, most heartily, into my desire for getting statistics from the different townships and parts of townships. He accordingly obtained lists of all the deaths by consumption, and calculated the relative population by the number of scholars in thirteen distinctly different districts in Townsend, where he then resided. These data were thrown together in one mass, those of the wet, medium and dry districts being promiscuously mingled. The materials were, in fact, chaotic in their unarranged details. I looked in vain, for some time, for any thread to guide me through the labyrinth of facts. Finally, I threw the letter aside, fearing that though there were facts enough, I should make little of them. As I have hinted above, at the time of receiving them, I had no idea of the existence of any law, in any degree, regulating the production of consumption, within *very limited districts.* With entire scepticism as to the result, I finally, months subsequently to my first reception of them, again took up these data, intending to classify, if possible, the thirteen districts according to the relative amounts of moisture in the soil in each. In order to prevent entirely any bias being given to my mind from vague notions I had already gained of the influence of this law of soil moisture in the State at large, I covered from sight the mortuary statistics, while I was classifying the districts. They could be arranged as follows, viz:—1, dry; 2, "hills, with clayey subsoil, retaining moisture;" 3, "near damp spots;" 4, "in wet and low places." Now, gentlemen, I can assure you that, when on examination of the record of deaths, I *found such an exact relation to exist* in all the four classes of districts *between the amount of soil-dampness and the number of deaths by consumption*, I was beyond measure surprised. I seemed on the point of finding out one of the, hitherto unnoticed, laws of development of this dire scourge of our race, and by attention to which, we might hope for some future alleviation of it. For *did not these facts, as far as one imperfeet series of facts could do so, seem to indicate that consumption varies immensely with the character of the soil, even within very narrow limits ?*

When I revolved in my mind the possibility of this being an exact representation of a great truth, and then thought of the vast influence the thorough knowledge of it must have upon our professional practice, and of the beneficial effects upon Public Hygiene that would perhaps result, *in future*, from an intelligent obedience to it by the community at large, it was the happiest and most satisfactory moment of my professional life. I remembered that over twenty thousand* consumptive patients had died in Massachusetts during the previous five years. I asked myself these questions :—Supposing this township represents the various townships of the State, and that they all have their varieties of soil, then if this township's statistics are true, and at least twice as many die in the wet as in the dry districts, may not similar results have occurred and perhaps be still occurring all over the State in which these twenty thousand human beings have been slain? Having arrived at this point, you will not be surprised at my asking, still further, this pregnant question :—If our fathers and we had paid greater attention to

* In Registration Report, 1857, we find that during the five years, including 1853 to '57, 23,280 died of consumption in Massachusetts.

this law, and we had always resided in dry localities, leaving the lower and moister for the purposes of business, perhaps, during the day, or for agriculture, should we not be saving over one thousand lives annually in Massachusetts, which are now foolishly sacrificed? These questions I then answered but imperfectly, but statistics since received, and of which I shall hereafter give you, I hope, more convincing examples, have only made me, each year, more firm in the conviction of the affirmative of these questions, at least in all their essential elements.

I pass, however, now to my fourth line of evidence.

IV.—Peculiarities of certain Villages in certain Townships, in one of which Consumption is quite prevalent, and in another much less so, these appearances being connected most closely with corresponding differences in the amount of moisture of the soil and exposure of said Villages.

I have only two townships of which the resident physicians have given me statistics, each of two villages within their own immediate circle of practice, and concerning which they are thoroughly acquainted. These townships are Marlboro' and West Boylston.

The former, twenty-five miles west of Boston, is one of the best agricultural towns in the State. Dr. E. T. Barnes thus describes two villages: Both are situated higher than the adjacent towns; both have a strong loamy soil, rocky, full of springs, and both seem equal in this respect. The more westerly one is one hundred and fifty to two hundred and fifty feet higher than the other. It runs north and south upon a ridge of hills, which ridge is the first obstacle the gusts and blasts from Wachusett and Monadnock Mountains meet with, in their career from north-west to south-east. They rush over this village with the greatest violence and velocity. The east village, running east and west, is sheltered on the west, north and east by considerable hills, and is comparatively exempt from these inconveniences. The snow remains much longer in the former than in the latter. The town contains more than 4200 inhabitants, and Dr. Barnes can remember all who have died of phthisis during the last ten years. He says forty, or perhaps one or two more, are all who have died of consumption in the township, during that period. Of these, eighteen were residents in the more exposed village; three or four resided in the least exposed village. This statement, of course, simply asserts, that of two equally damp villages, that which has the bleaker exposure has suffered more from consumption than the other that is less exposed. It is, therefore, another argument that consumption is not equally prevalent in every part of the State; but proves nothing in regard to dampness alone. While claiming dampness of the soil as *one of the prime causes of consumption in New England, I do not assert that it is the sole cause, or that the combination of changeableness and coldness with moisture, may not be vastly more fatal than moisture alone.*

The statistics of the second town, viz., West Boylston, is definitely in favor of dampness as a cause of consumption, while at the same time they suggest the importance of defence from the northern and eastern blasts.

Dr. Lovell, the resident physician, gave me such a deeply interesting account of the differences between the two villages, in their relative amount of pulmonary disease, that I was induced to visit them.

I found them as follows: In the village where consumption prevails, the houses are situated nearly on the immediate level of a mill-pond, and at the junction of two rivers. Water seems permeating every where, and not a cellar, as it seemed to me, can escape its influence. To increase the coldness of the spot, the north and north-east winds have full access to it through the river valley. Although the day was fair and not at all cold, I felt chilly as I drove through it. Dr. Lovell assures me that the nights in this village are cool and damp, seldom without a fog. The other village, a mile or more distant, is situated on a ridge of land, fifty or sixty feet above a small artificial pond, surrounded chiefly by a sandy beach. North of the village, but at a certain distance from it, arises a high ridge of sandy hills, covered with woods. The whole position is evidently one entirely different from that of the other village, being essentially dry, warm, open to the genial southern sun, and defended from northern and eastern blasts. Dr. Lovell says: "The air here is generally warm and dry, so that the inhabitants sleep with their windows open from early spring to late in the autumn." Dr. Lovell gave me statistics for 15 years, and the estimated relative population of the two villages, viz., 500 in the moister and colder, and 200 in the drier and warmer. In the former he had had 12 cases of consumption, in the latter only 1. He had likewise noticed a much greater prevalence of other diseases, connected with the air-passages, as croup and bronchitis, pneumonia, &c. in the damper village. At the time of my visit, I observed with painful anticipations, that low down on the very edge of the pond, at the base of the bluff on which the drier village stands, and over almost the only land, that presented a wet, meadowy aspect, the proprietor of the factory was erecting a new building, for the purpose of using it as a residence for his workmen, nearer to their place of work than the houses, on the ridge above. I even then feared the result, and I beg you to mark the fact that has since occurred, I will not say, in consequence, but certainly in connection with this change of location of the residences of the people, viz.: Dr. Lovell remarked to me within the past year, that, since his first report to me in 1855 and '56, consumption had appeared to be more prevalent in that village.

V. — Certain Houses, which, in various Towns, have been long known, by the inhabitants and by Resident Physicians, as the abodes of Consumptive Patients, and in some of which, several families have been, during the past fifty years, cut off by Consumption.

The evidence I shall present upon this point and during the remainder of these remarks, I have never placed before you at any previous period, they having been all procured since my report in 1856. They are among the most remarkable I have obtained. By them I think I shall lead you very strongly to suspect, even if I do not wholly convince you, that this all-powerful law of soil-moisture exerts its baleful influences within still narrower compass, than any previously hinted at, and that *even some houses may become the foci of consumption, when others but slightly removed from them, but on a drier soil, almost wholly escape.*

I am myself acquainted with two houses within twelve miles of Boston, in which I have no doubt this influence is working. I almost daily saw one while erecting by a speculator, at the very mouth of a low valley, running directly into Charles River, and but a foot or two above the level of the water. On each side of this valley arise high and sandy hills. With each evening sunset, a flood of cold moisture, almost if not quite imperceptible to eyesight, but quite palpable to the sensitive skin of the traveller, settles in between the hills and gradually envelops this devoted house. I have often passed the spot late at night. At times the moon shone clearly on the immediately adjacent ridges, but as I descended from them and passed the house, the rays were obscured, and a chilly feeling came over me, as if taking a cold bath. On these occasions I thought that if there were any truth in this apparent law of soil-moisture, I should hear of its effects on the family residing there. During the first year of their residence, the father suffered with a low and chronic cachexia. About two years afterwards, the wife consulted me for a cough, that had been coming on insidiously for several months. She was not of a consumptive family. I was not surprised, though certainly shocked, at finding, in addition to rational signs, undoubted crepitus under the left clavicle. I prescribed the usual remedies for early phthisis, but I felt bound then, and have no reason to doubt that the advice was strictly correct, to say that the *first* thing to be done, if safety was to be gained for the patient, was her immediate and permanent change of location to some dry, neighboring hill, or still better, to some place, more thoroughly removed from any dampness. My advice came too late.

I beg you to understand that I do not present this by itself as any proof that dampness of location produces consumption. In this case it may be, and doubtless many of you think it is, a mere coincidence. I have no right, perhaps, to object to that view. *I have, however, had too many of such coincidences.* They, as it were, simply compose the *complement* of the general evidence to the existence of the law. I therefore regard this one case as more significant than most of you perhaps will, at present, allow.

Let us proceed. I know another homestead in which resides a family of wealth and refinement. It is a sweet rural cottage, overhung with clustering vines, delightfully situated amid shade trees, thickly hemmed in "by a shrubberry that Shenstone might have envied." It rests on the borders of a sylvan lake, on a rich, loamy, fertile, moist soil, a few feet only from the water, and scarcely more than a few inches above its level. In the heats of our midsummer, every passer-by would point out the spot, as one to be selected for its perfect coolness of situation and quiet loveliness. But I fear it is most unhealthy, and for the following reason. The parents occupying it, are themselves healthy, and have had ten children. None have been perfectly robust. Three have already died of consumption. A fourth has it now, in its last stages. The young daughters who remain are, during the day time, some miles away at school, in a high and dry location. They sleep at home. They do not seem so strong as others, and in the eyes of neighbors seem threatened with the disease of which the others died. One son, who is constantly at sea, is healthy.

A previous occupant of this house died of consumption. His family was liable to frequent coughs, while resident there, from which they have escaped since their removal.

All this has happened, and yet I cannot persuade the parents that the pleasant house, in its present location, is the charnel-house of their race, as I verily believe it to be.

Again, pass with me into the interior of the State, and visit another town, very undulating, chiefly agricultural, with one small village, through which runs a stream, between abrupt hills. This place I visited the past summer, in order to see three or four houses, that had been brought to my notice by Dr. Lyman Bartlett, of New Bedford, as proving the truth of the views I have endeavored to bring before you. It was his native place, and he knew whereof he spoke. No less than three houses he alluded to, as having been nests of consumption. One has only to see them to perceive how entirely their position supports our general views. Two of them are in a low, narrow valley, hidden from the sun by lofty and luxuriantly growing shade trees. The soil, on which they rest, is bursting with moisture, and close by, that is, within a few feet of each, is a mill-stream or pond, the waters from which keep the foundations of the houses perpetually bathed with moisture. Of these I shall forbear here to speak,* but will enter more into detail about a third — the story of which may be told by the following summary:

1. Four grandparents lived to a healthy old age, and died over eighty years old. One of the grandmothers always bore on her neck, scars, said to be from scrofulous ulcers in early life.

2. Two brothers, A and B, married two sisters, both couples being children of these grandparents. All parties were in perfect health at the time of marriage, and with no thought of consumption ever entering their families.

3. After his marriage, A staid in the old homestead, situated on a southern slope, a dry and warm, well-drained spot, where he was born, and there all his children were born and reared to adult life.

B, on the contrary, moved to a house subjected to wholly different influences, and there his children were born and reared to adult life.†

---

* See Appendix D, for the details.

† The diagram annexed presents the place more distinctly than any mere description. In a few words, it may be said to be situated in a wholly

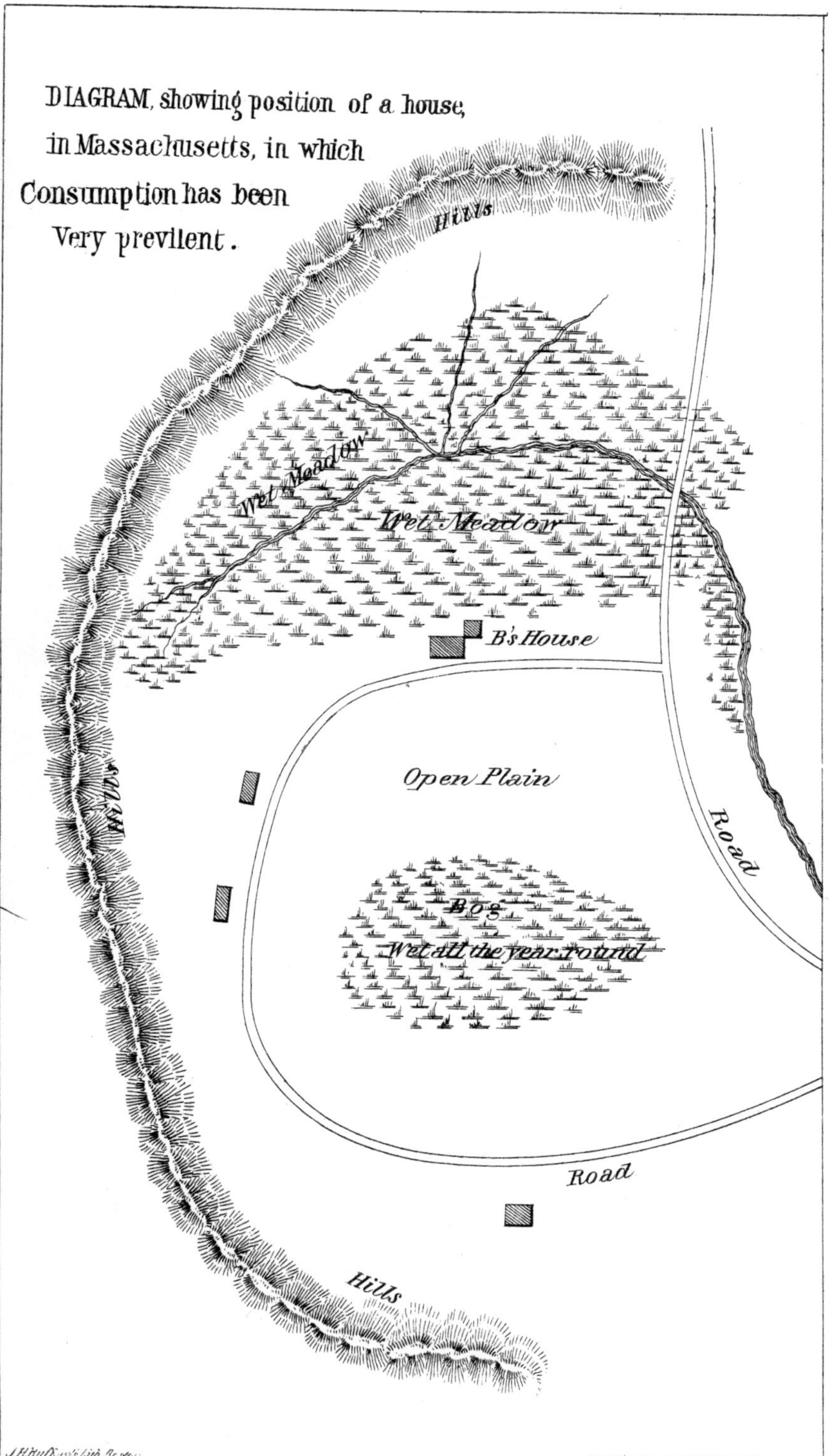
DIAGRAM, showing position of a house, in Massachusetts, in which Consumption has been Very previlent.
Hills
Wet Meadow
Wet Meadow
B's House
Open Plain
Road
Bog
Wet all the year round
Road
Hills
Hills
Consumption in Massachusetts

The subsequent results in the two families are clearly shown in the subjoined table:

No. Persons in Families A & B.		Now Alive.		Died.						Total Deaths in Family.
Parents.	Children.	In good health.	Consumptive Cough.	Consumption.	Scrofulous Swellings.	Acute Brain Disease.	Acute Bowel Disease.	Diabetes.	Croup.	
A, 2	9	6	....	....	1 quite yg.	1 æt.25	1	....	....	3
B, 2	11	3*	1	6 child.	....	....	....	1	1	9
....	....	....	....	Mother, æt. 63.	....	...	...	....	....	....

* Father and two sons; the sons having been away from home many years.

The statement of the two families may be made briefly as follows:—Both families, as we have seen, had by one grandmother slight tendencies to scrofula, although consumption proper had never entered into the known tendencies of any ancestor. This was, in fact, a strong belief in the minds of both families.

Of thirteen persons (parents and children), in family B, nine have died; seven (more than two thirds of them), *by consumption;* one of croup, and one of diabetes. Of the surviving four (father and three children), one has been for years slowly *suffering* from apparently *pulmonary disease.* The three others, namely, father and two sons, are healthy; but these two sons have not lived in the homestead for many years. On the contrary, of the eleven persons (parents and children) in family A, three have died

different spot. Low, with hills closely surrounding it; a wet meadow comes up directly to the cellar wall; a bog, wet all the year, is in front; a river is hard by. Moisture is the principal characteristic of the surroundings of the house.

(less than one third), and not one has died of *consumption*, though one died early with scrofula.

The skeptic will shake his knowing head and ask again, What does one example of this kind prove? In answer, I would ask whether, if the objector should find his own family dying around him by the same disease, under like circumstances, and should happen to have read the various correspondence and gained even the meagre, as he might deem them, statistical data I have presented, he would not then deem it the part of prudence to take it for granted that the fate of his wife and children looked very much like an illustration of the law? Whether this be admitted or not, I contend that, until the State or another individual has, by an overwhelming accumulation of evidence, refuted, what they may deem, my small proof, no physician or father ought to dare to neglect the evidence I have, even thus far, laid before him from educated physicians of Massachusetts; and among other data, he should weigh these examples.

I pass over Medway, Pembroke, Tewksbury, Sudbury*—in all of which are found cases of a similar, though perhaps less marked character, and shall close this part of my subject with the following statement, eminently illustrative of the truth of the law we are discussing. It shows also how this law has been acting for years, is acting now, probably not only in the township I shall name, but likewise in various other places in this Commonwealth—while the public, and attending physicians sit by, ignoring

---

* See Appendix D, for details.

its fatal tendencies, and allowing family after family to be cut down by residing where, I verily believe, God never meant that man should live and attempt to rear a family.

Many years ago, and before I had arrived at definite conclusions on this subject, I was visiting Franklin, Mass., on professional business, and I asked the physician whether "any portion of his town was peculiarly liable to consumption." His prompt response was "Nay." In a few moments, however, and in continuation of the subject suggested by the question, he said—"But I wish you would explain why three houses in this town have been famed for having had consumptive families in them."

Avoiding carefully all leading questions, and especially any allusion to the vague notions in regard to the influence of soil I then held, I desired him to make a rough drawing of the position of the houses, and to tell me the characters of the soil, on which they were built, and of the vicinity. I give a copy of that drawing in the subjoined diagram.

The houses A B C could not be situated in a position more favorable for an "*experimentum crucis*" of this law, supposing it to exist. Exposed to the north and east, their foundations rest on a soil permeated with water; the base of the hill, on which they stand, being skirted by meadow and pond, so that every north-east wind comes freighted with moisture upon them. Even the warm and genial sun strikes the hill at an angle, and as it were slides *over* rather than lights upon it, not penetrating, as when the rays strike at right angles to the surface of the soil. Listen to the tale told by these tenements.

In one (A), formerly resided a woman who had been born on the estate.* She married, and had five children. The husband and all but one of the children sickened and died of consumption. The one surviving child became very feeble, took alarm, suspected the locality, moved away to what he deemed a more healthy location, recovered his health, and is now enjoying a green, healthy old age of upwards of 70 years.

Thus much for the history of this house, previous to the present occupants taking possession of it. These present occupants are not as healthy as farmers and their families usually are. The father has had hæmoptysis several times. The daughter has pains in her back, shoulder and sides of chest, and is under medical care. One son is like this sister. One son is healthy.

The second house, B. Parents and grandparents healthy. Parents have lived here twenty years. Eldest daughter bled—left home and gained in health; returned and died of consumption, October, 1855. Second daughter always at home; died of consumption in 1853. Third daughter has cough, is feeble, and unable to attend school in consequence; is, in the opinion of her physician, a doomed girl, to die of consumption. Fourth daughter, aged 22, has pains in her side; works irregularly; her physician is apprehensive of her. A son had cough at the

* She had five brothers or sisters, all of whom removed from the homestead, and no consumption appeared among them.

DIAGRAM, showing position of three houses placed on a hill in Mass. in which for 50 past years, consumption has been very previlent. a,b,c,d, outline of base of hill.

A,B, C, houses.

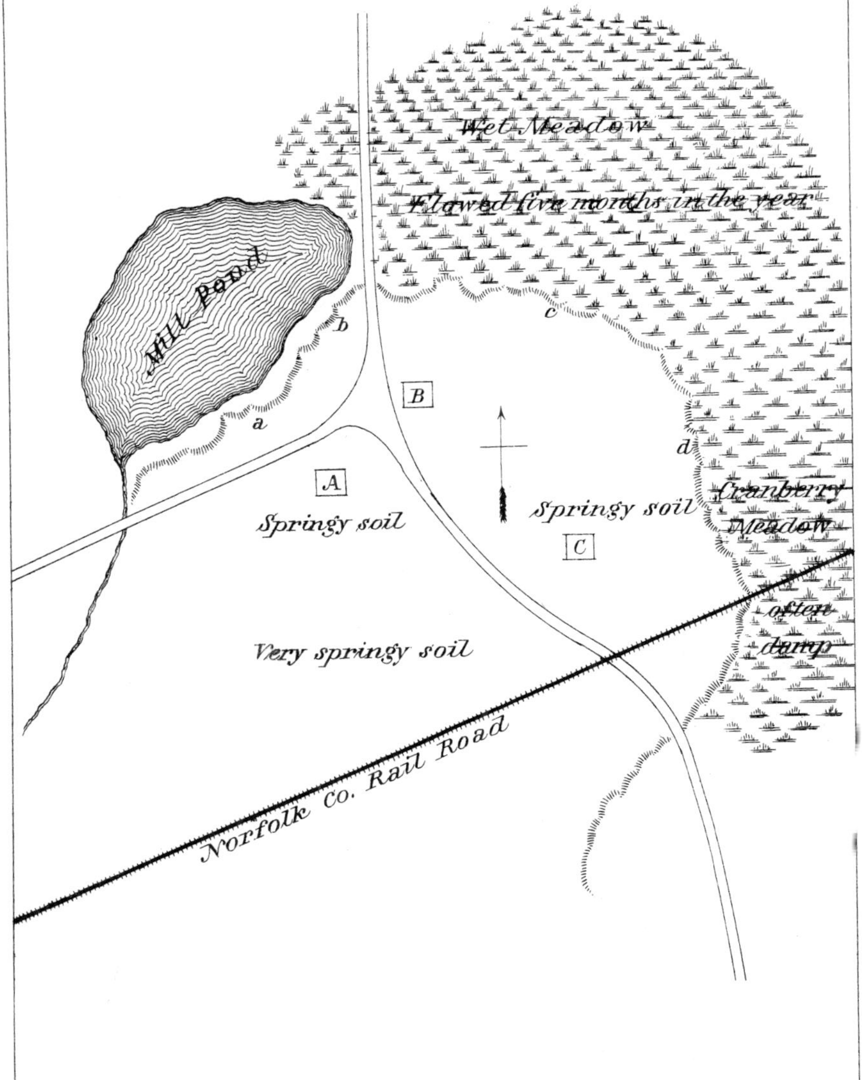

J.H. Bufford's Lith. Boston.

old homestead; he left and has improved his health. Second son, 18 years old, with depressed chest; weakly; left home and became better. On returning home, he became worse, and observed that, from *some* cause, he was not so well, felt less buoyant at home than in Vermont. Third son, 8 years old; a pale, sickly child.

The third house, C. Former occupants, parents healthy. Two children died of consumption, one of scrofula.

Present occupants, less healthy than other families in different parts of the town. Father, rheumatic; mother, healthy; one daughter died of consumption, one of scrofula; a son became deaf at eighteen or twenty years of age.

What think you of the illustration? Look distinctly at the facts. Of 14 grandparents and parents, 12 were said to have been healthy. Of the remaining 2, 1 has had hæmoptysis; 1 is rheumatic.

Of 21 children, only 2 have been healthy. Of the remaining 19, 9 have died of consumption; 2 of scrofula; 7 are sickly and weak, or evidently affected with pulmonary disease; 1 is deaf.

Why are so many sick? Why so many dead? Why cannot the children live well at their own homes? I attribute it to the location. If you had had half the evidence I have now given to prove that a damp soil is one of the great causes of consumption in Massachusetts, and it had been applicable to diseases of an intermittent type — fever and ague, for example — you would have had no doubt about the question, but would have instantly declared the tenements unhealthy. But you doubt, perhaps, in regard to consumption, because it is not one of the medical dogmas of the times that consumption has any local origin, of such a nature as, I think, I have exhibited to you.

Having thus given you some facts, collected in Massachusetts, I pass now to: —

VI. — Confirmatory Opinions, Facts and Statistics, from Rhode Island, Maine and New Hampshire.

I have obtained returns from ten towns without the limits of the State; viz., from Maine, New Hampshire and Rhode Island. They amply support the views already presented. Briefly given, the reports from these towns are as follows:

Dr. Trafton, of Kennebunk Port, Maine, assures me that consumption is much more rife at the Port, where there is a clayey, moist soil and a coast exposure, than at Kennebunk itself — a fine township, higher, chiefly sandy, with many pine woods, and few, if any, meadows — precisely, in fact, those differences which, I am led to think, will often, hereafter, be found to exist between spots suffering in different degrees from consumption.

Dr. T. also assured me that a house, whose cellar wall is washed daily by the incoming tide (being built directly upon a creek, connected with the ocean), has been the residence of a family, every member of which, except the parents, *have been born and reared, and have died of consumption, in that place.*

The childless parents have now moved away, in their old age, only to let another younger couple beget another puny set of children, as those already born are now becoming. Dr. T. mentioned this house to me, in answer to my question whether any household in his town was peculiarly troubled by consumption; and I judged from his remark, that, although he, doubtless, would not have chosen the place as a healthy location, he did not put the location and consumption as cause and effect — which *I* verily did.

Dr. Marrett, of Saccarappa, near Portland, gives the following statistics, on his own and Dr. Stone's practice.

Dr. Marrett says, "The whole town, with few exceptions, possesses a cold, wet and clayey loam soil." The "plain district has more of a dry, gravelly soil."

Dr. M.'s statistics of his own practice in the whole town, for eight years, 1842 to 1851, were as follows: All deaths, 66; by consumption, 21 — or 31.81 per cent.

Dr. Stone's statistics of his own practice, during the same period, for the whole town, were as follows: All deaths, 104; by consumption, 32 — or 30.76 per cent. In the "plain district" he had: All deaths, 68; by consumption, 11—or 16.17 per cent.

These data are in complete analogy with the statistics of Townsend, West Newbury, &c., in Massachusetts.

Dr. Allen, of Saco, Maine, than whom there lives no more intelligent witness — a practitioner of long standing — assures me that, in his own practice, for fifteen years past, he has noticed that, on two ridges of land, whose only difference consists of this characteristic of moisture of the soil, almost every family has been decimated on the wet part, while almost all upon the dry portion have escaped. This statement is a most striking exemplification of the views already given. It seems likewise to show that it is not *elevation* or *exposure*, or a certain amount of cultivation or woodland, nor any peculiar trade, &c., that is the cause of the malady; for, in all these respects, the two localities seem alike. One ridge is quite dry, the other is literally filled with springs. Nowhere can a spade be driven a few feet into the ground, without meeting water. In fact, in former times, the superstitious frequently had their friends, who had died of consumption, disinterred, and Dr. Allen invariably found the coffins filled with water, however shallow may have been the graves.

Dr. Sanborn, of Hampton Falls, N. H., gives statistics of that town and of old Hampton, which, at first sight, seem to give little support to my views. But I find, on accurate analysis of the returns, that in Hampton, two thirds of all the cases of consumption occurred on a ridge of land, nearer to the marshes, and where one fifth only of the inhabitants live.

So, at Hampton Falls: the inhabited part, that is, the dampest, has twice as many consumptive cases, in proportion to the population, as the driest and highest.

At Newport, N. H., Dr. Richardson speaks of two houses near a mill pond, and around which runs a river, the entire soil being thus made very moist. The parents, three children and a stranger lady, resident in the family, have died of consumption within four years. *A remaining son and daughter moved away to a drier location, remained cachectic for some time, and have finally recovered* — an example wholly analogous to what we have noticed at Franklin, Mass. How long will you shut your eyes to these facts, and your intellects to their importance, in your daily practice ?

Drs. Hartwell and Tuttle, report from Farmington, N.H. Dr. Tuttle says the town is on low, moist land. He and Dr. Hartwell have both noticed that consumption is much more prevalent there than on the surrounding hills. Dr. H., from eighteen months statistics, gives as the number of deaths by all diseases, 43 ; of which 13 were by consumption—or 30.23 per cent.

Dr. Clough, of Greenland, has a town singularly but very distinctly marked by three classes of soil, viz., 1st, a higher, drier, sandy plain ; 2d, a medium, fertile, rather moist portion ; 3d, extensive low marshes. I asked for statistics, and he returns these : Population, 715, about equally divided in the districts ; families, 150. During 10 years, 1847 to 1857, 3 persons died in the dry district, 5 in the medium, and 10 in the wet. Small statistics, but significant !

Dr. Hovey, of Atkinson, N. H. It is a dry, well-drained township, sloping very gradually to those adjacent to it. The first thought of Dr. Hovey was, that the statistics of the town, in which he was born and had resided, and had practised medicine nearly fifty years, would not sustain the views submitted in this report. I begged for statistics, as I knew that he was acquainted with all the townspeople who had died. From the general characteristics of the town, I thought there would be but few cases of consumption in it. I was in doubt whether the law of dampness, acting so slightly as I thought it must, would show itself with sufficient distinctness.

Dr. H. writes, from a review of thirty years, and informs me, while giving the data, that he is convinced, that, though very small, they fully sustain the influence of dampness of locality as productive of consumption. Population, 606. Total deaths, 203; by consumption, 40. In driest districts, one died of consumption in every 56 persons; in medium districts, one in 15.50; in wet, one in 5. The proportion of deaths by consumption to total deaths, he found as follows: 9.75 in the high and dry, 17.64 in the medium, and 50.00 in the low districts.

Dr. Ellis, of Bristol, Rhode Island, has noticed that few persons are affected with consumption in Bristol, compared with the number found in Warren, a few miles distant. Bristol stands on a bold, rocky shore, washed by the waves of a bay, opening upon the Atlantic. It is defended somewhat, at the east, by a line of hills. Warren, on the contrary, is situated low, on the wet land adjacent to the marshes of the bay. The higher tides are apt to overflow them, at times, quite up to the borders of the town. There is, moreover, no defence from the cold easterly winds. It

DIAGRAM, showing relative position of BRISTOL to WARREN, R.I.

From a Sketch, by Dr. J. James Ellis.

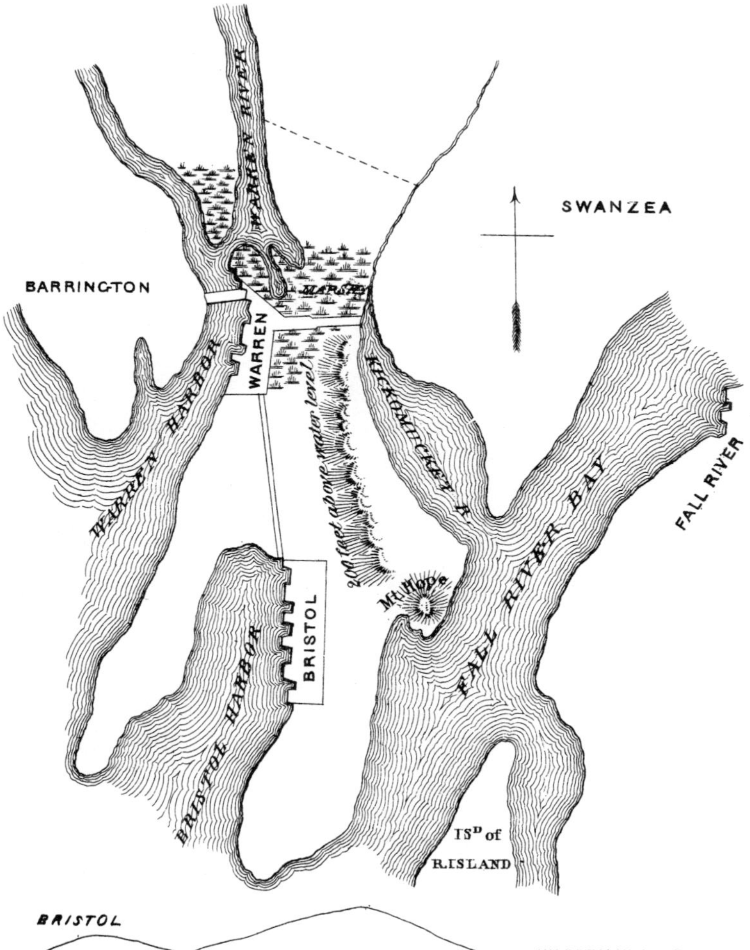

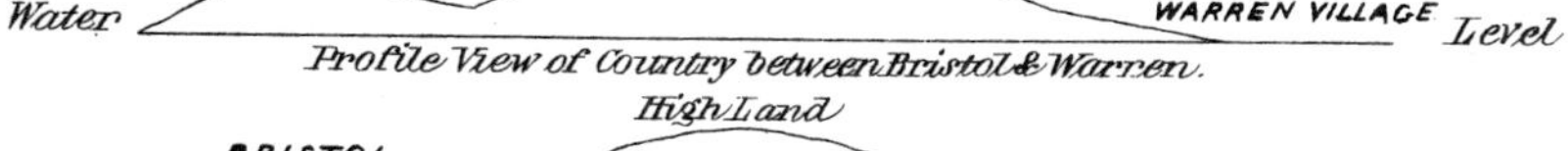

Profile View of Country between Bristol & Warren.

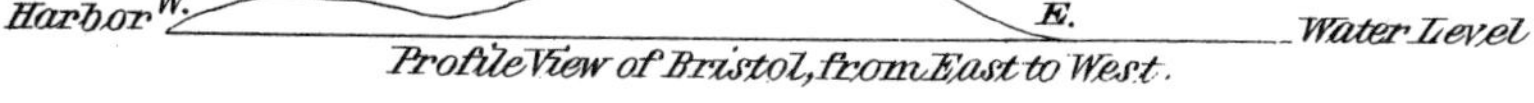

Profile View of Bristol, from East to West.

J.H. Bufford's Lith. Boston.

is but right to say, that the Rhode Island State Registration Report for 1859 throws some doubt on this statement of Dr. E. That of 1860, however, shows there is an unequal distribution of consumption in the various counties of the State.

May I not say that these data from Maine, New Hampshire and Rhode Island, afford nearly as certain evidence of the operation of this law of dampness throughout New England, as we have for its prevalence in Massachusetts? *A priori*, we must admit that *any* etiological climate-law, acting in Massachusetts, must extend over the New England States, so entirely analogous are they in their characteristics.

But if it extend over New England, an interesting question immediately arises, whether the same influence is spread over the United States. To decide what is public opinion or fact on this subject, I shall appeal to Drs. Forry, Drake, Blodgett, Lawson, and Coolidge, in his United States Army Report.

Dr. Forry* does not believe in moisture as the cause of consumption, nor that cold, *per se*, is necessarily so. I have the highest respect for Dr. Forry, as an able pioneer in the climatology of the United States; but the subject of soil-moisture, as the cause of consumption, was really never thoroughly discussed by him, as we are now able to reason upon it, from the returns made by the Massachusetts Medical Society.

* The Climate of the United States and its Endemic Influences. By Samuel Forry, M.D. New York: I. & H. G. Langley. 1846.

Dr. Drake,* one of the most vigorous minds and original writers of our profession, enters extensively into the topic, but he cannot grapple with it, as we are able, with our facts, to do. He doubts the effect of humidity, as a cause of consumption. He believes in a dry, cold climate as being rather unlikely to cause it. In this, we certainly agree. He certainly disbelieves the views often entertained, that a cold climate necessarily causes it. He thinks, and I presume all the profession will agree with him, that damp, unventilated apartments are bad for consumptive patients. But you see that he really hardly touches our topic.

Mr. Blodgett† (p. 474) comes nearer to our view when he says of "*climate*," "dry and warm are required for the relief or cure of pulmonary disease." Again: "In warm, very variable, with much humidity, the requisite conditions are wanting." And finally, he enumerates what is perfectly true: "*Dry* (his own italics) and equable districts are the great desideratum, though, in humid and equable climates, it is far less frequently induced than in cold and humid."

Dr. Lawson,‡ in his admirable work on Phthisis (page 241), takes the ground that moisture is a comparatively unimportant agent in the production of phthisis. But he does not really treat our subject,

---

* The Principal Diseases of the Interior Valley of North America. Second Series, &c. Philadelphia: Lippincott, Grambo & Co. 1854.

† Climatology of the United States. By Lorin Blodgett. Philadelphia: Lippincott, Grambo & Co. 1857.

‡ A Practical Treatise on Phthisis Pulmonalis. By L. M. Lawson, M.D. Cincinnati and New York: S. S. & W. Wood. 1861.

viz., the damp soil. He speaks of circumambient atmosphere, amount of rain, &c. But it is evident that Pau, for example, which has much rain, but whose atmosphere is, really, generally dry, owing to the quick absorption of rain by the porous soil, is very differently situated, and may be much drier, and better for a consumptive patient than another spot, where the soil or subsoil is perpetually filled with inherent moisture, and but very little rain falls.

But the most important, and by far the most satisfactory statements in favor of my general views, may be found in Dr. Coolidge's most admirable Reports of the Medical Statistics of the United States Army. To this I now call attention.

VII.—Medical Statistics, given in the Report on the Health of the United States Army; intimating the existence of this Law and of its wide operation over the whole of this Continent, contained within the limits of the United States.

Dr. Coolidge* has made the most valuable report, ever published on this continent, on the health of the soldier in different parts of our country. In reference to the subject in which we feel most interested, I quote the following very valuable opinion, as actu-

* Statistical Report on the Sickness and Mortality in the Army of the United States, compiled from the Records of the Surgeon-General's Office, embracing a period of sixteen years, from January, 1839, to January, 1855. Prepared under direction of Brevet Brigadier Gen. Thomas Lawson, Surg. Gen., by Richard H. Coolidge, M.D., Ass't Surg. U. S. A. Washington, 1856. Also Second Report, from 1855 to '59.

ally deductions from facts observed. In the text I shall give only summaries, and refer the reader to the Appendix* for more and very interesting details on this topic.

After premising that it may be generally considered of doubtful propriety for a compiler to present his own individual inferences, but that, in regard to the amount and ratio of phthisis in the several regions, he feels called upon not to adhere to his original intention of being simply a compiler, he makes the following statements in his first report (p. 497):

"The most important atmospherical condition for a consumptive is DRYNESS." * * * "Next to DRY is an EQUABLE temperature." * * "A uniformly *low* is better than a uniformly *high* temperature." "The worst possible climate for a consumptive is one with long-continued high temperature and high dew point."

So, too, if we examine particular facts, given in his second report, they are eminently significant.

Assistant Surgeon Robert Bartholow writes (p. 306), March, 1859, from Fort Bridger, in Utah, "in the upper cold regions," "very dry" atmosphere, soil of valley "light, porous, sandy, through which the water percolates constantly:"

"The most interesting fact with regard to the influence of this climate upon the thoracic affections, is the amelioration and cure of pulmonary, tubercular disease. Not a single case of phthisis has occurred at this post, and those, who came here laboring

* Appendix F.

under the symptoms more or less advanced, are notably improved."

Assistant Surgeon Basil Norris writes, from Fort Clark, Texas, September, 1856: The Fort "is situated on a healthy site, overlooking the surrounding country. It has a *dry* and equable climate." "Pulmonary diseases are rare. The dry and equable climate has been beneficial to a few cases left in the hospital, and at the post none have originated." —(p. 190.)

Similar remarks are made by Ass't Surg. Robert Bartholow on Camp Scott, in Utah (p. 291). "All who came hither, laboring under the incipient or well-established symptoms of consumption, speedily improved." The dryness and equableness of the climate is noted as the most important element in the cure. Conjoined with this, however, were improved hygiene, and mountain height.

From the above, am I not allowed to suspect that the law of moisture of the soil as the cause of consumption prevails in other parts of the United States more generally than in New England?

Does this Law hold good in other parts of the World?

In order to show more precisely the facts, in regard to the dampness or dryness of various places, and their reputed influence on phthisis, I have endeavored to obtain the characteristics of the soils of various places named, as peculiarly advantageous for phthisical patients, as given by Sir James Clarke, Messrs. I. P. Knox, Dix, Henry Rhind, Alexander Taylor,

Dr. Burgess, John McClelland, James R. Martin, C. R. Hall, Twining, Beddoes, Walter S. Baker, Dr. Jourdant, Lawson, Mühry, Boudin, Poissac and Lombard, writers that treat of all the climates of the known globe. I found as follows:

Places, of whose soil I can find any sufficient account, and which are said to be good for consumptive patients as residences; for example: Pau, Villa-Franca, Malta, Madeira, Canary Islands, Azores, Bermudas, Bahamas, Undercliff, St. Croix, St. Thomas, Egypt, Nice, Mexico, Algiers, have essentially dry soils, and, though some have great rains, the atmospherical surroundings of the patient become rapidly dry, even after rain.

Others, such as Pisa, Naples, Milan, Parma, Mantua, Verona, Exmouth, Sidmouth, all said to be prejudicial to consumptives, have essentially moist soils.

Notwithstanding all this, Mühry,* one of the ablest of European writers, doubts the influences of moisture; but he has no facts, strictly speaking, bearing upon our precise question.

Boudin,† also, an equally great writer on this subject, still holds to the opinion that moist, intermittent fever countries prevent phthisis.

Dr. Lombard,‡ of Geneva, claims nothing for dryness as a preventive. But he and Mühry both

* Klimatologische Unstersuchungen, &c. A. Mühry. Leipsic and Heidelberg. 1858.

† Traité de Géographie et de Statistiques Medicales, &c. Par I. Ch. M. Boudin. Paris: Baillère. 1856.

‡ Les Climats des Montagnes, &c. H. C. Lombard, Geneva and Paris. Joel Cherbuliez. 1858.

assert that, at a certain height in the Swiss mountains (Mühry states the same of the whole globe), consumption is unknown. They attribute the fact to the rarefied air. I would claim much for the dryness, which necessarily accompanies the height.

The sum total of our investigations into European works is, that, while no writer attaches the same value to moisture of the soil, that I have been compelled to do, from my examination of New England, the fact that so large a proportion of places, famed for giving relief to consumptives, have dry soils, is, to use the mildest term, a peculiar coincidence.

I do not think, moreover, that the subject has ever been fairly investigated with reference to the influence of *soil-moisture* on the prevalence of consumption, as I have investigated it in these researches. In confirmation of this assertion, I would remark, that although I brought the subject (during a visit to Europe in 1859), as fully as I could before men of experience in vital statistics in England, and on the continent, I never found but one person who, practically, could give any evidence on the subject. This gentleman was a physician in the highlands of Scotland, whose name, I regret, has escaped me. He had practised in two valleys, one of which has a great deal of moist soil, and consumption is very prevalent there, while the other is much drier and has much less consumption. The physician had not apparently connected the two facts, in the relation of cause and effect.

VIII.—Results of my own Practice, since I first became convinced of the Truth of this Law.

(a) *Statistics from my private records of Cases.*

Out of 201 patients, from the country townships of New England, distinctly affected both with the rational and physical signs of consumption, such as distinct râles under the clavicle, &c., I find that 109, or more than one half, are reported to be residents *on* decidedly damp places, and one half of the remainder have lived in houses having damp cellars, or their houses are situated *near* damp localities. Thus *three quarters of all these patients* have resided, *where dampness of the soil is a prominent characteristic.* Somewhat less than one quarter resided in dry places.

(b) *Results of my Practice, when applying this Law to the Prevention or Cure of Consumption.*

Since I became convinced that a residence, on or near a damp locality, is actually promotive of consumption, I have acted fully up to that belief, and have had satisfactory results. The following statements I make deliberately, for they are true. The cases, to be alluded to, have been under my own care. I have seen whereof I speak, in every particular.

First. Persons having had hæmoptysis and irritation of the lungs, and who have apparently been threatened with phthisis, but without physical signs, have been completely restored to health, by changing their place of residence, according to the principles inculcated in this address, viz., by going to live in a dry locality, and leading more active lives. These patients have considered the change of location as the *prime* cause of their improved health, although I did not neglect other remedial measures. They perceived, moreover, the much greater balminess of the atmosphere, in its influence on their lungs, in these places, when compared not only with a city atmosphere, but with that in wet, country locations, very nearly adjacent to their own residences, equally beautiful to the eye, seeming, in fact, to the majority of persons, equally healthy. I am myself acquainted with two such spots, and the ascent of a long hill alone separates them. Doubtless, many of you have noticed similar differences in your own towns. Between the climatic influences of two such localities, when you drive through them, especially at night, when the caloric, luminous, and perhaps still more, the actinic rays of the sun are not shed upon either, these differences upon your healthy bodies appear immense. The two are no more comparable than the mild, equable, temperate atmosphere of a balmy day in September or October, and that we experience during the chilly north-east storms of early spring. Does it therefore seem incredible to you that such differences, even when not so appreciable during the waking hours, may materially influence our health during sleep, when our natures seem most susceptible of evil influences?

Second. I have had patients in whom physical signs of an undoubted character existed — such as crackling under the clavicle, diminished vesicular murmur, and some dulness on percussion—who, by removal from towns and localities lying under, or near, the influence of dampness of the soil, to another town very dry, have experienced immense benefit.

In one young lady, crackling disappeared almost wholly from the entire upper lobe of one lung, after a residence of six months in a very dry town, selected for the purpose, because the resident physician assured me that the town was very dry, and that cases of hæmoptysis that would, he thought, have terminated in fatal phthisis, in a town on the coast, where he previously resided, got well in his actual abode. The place was very different from the spot where she was taken ill, and where she resided, when I was first called to her, as hopelessly ill of hæmoptysis and consumption. And yet, were I to show you that very homestead, you would say it was one of the loveliest possible, with its long avenue of wide-spreading trees, on luxuriantly fertile soil; its quaint and picturesque, ancient architecture, indicating apparently that it had been the abode of many generations of families, of refined tastes and ample fortunes. Nevertheless, should you enter it at midday, at the hottest and most sultry hour in August, it would be like entering a cellar. I visited it, panting with the heat of a summer's sun. In a half hour I spent there, I was so chilled that I quickly sought, on going out, the genial influence of the same sun, I had, previously, gladly escaped from, in order to overcome a certain depressing coldness, that painfully affected me. This was the most remarkable case I ever had. The lady was subsequently married and lived a few years, and finally died of phthisis, under the following circumstances. Having got nearly, if not quite well, she begged, after many months residence at the selected spot, that she might be allowed to come nearer to the city, for the sake of her husband's business. In vain I protested. She, however, decided to remove, and although healthy sites were chosen in the country, ten miles from Boston, none were so dry as that first selected. Gradually, the cough returned, and fatal phthisis was the result.

I have no doubt, however, that life was prolonged by the first change. I think that had she remained at the place at which I first visited her, she would soon have died; and that if she had remained at the place which I chose for her, and where she so rapidly improved, she might be now alive.

I have had other cases of a similar nature, in which the rational signs were very threatening, with slight but unequivocal physical signs. In these, both classes of signs have disappeared under a change of place and rational treatment—the change, however, being deemed an essential element in the treatment, and, in my opinion, the most important part of it.

Third. I have had another and equally significant class of cases, in which undoubted and more extensive rational and physical signs of consumption have existed for a year or more, and in whom, even now, the physical signs are sufficiently well marked, though showing less irritation of the lungs; while the constitutional symptoms are very much better, under similar changes of residence.

In this catalogue are two married ladies, who, for years, have lived in a spot chosen by me because of the dryness of its soil, its elevation above the surrounding country, and its exposure towards the southern sun. These have been ill for several years, and had been so, when I first saw them. Both were living in damp localities; both moved to the place thus chosen, and there they established their family abodes. They have never had a desire for any permanent change. Both, it is true, have occasionally gone south. They both recognize and value the difference of effect upon their own lungs, between the air in the spot selected, and any other they may be called upon to breathe. Especially do they now feel the difference, in this respect, between their present location and the wet, meadowy abodes, in which they formerly resided, and where some of their friends now live.

To sum up the results of my experience, and my present judgment, on this subject, as a matter of therapeutics—I dare not neglect the abundant evidence of the influence of locality, as a cause of phthisis. Deeming it, in fact, one of the great causes of consumption in New England, I, of course, think of it in every case I meet with, and make it a rule to endeavor to learn, more precisely than I formerly did, the nature of the soil on or near which my patient is situated, and especially its character as to dryness or moisture, to which, when at home or on business, he is habitually subjected. If I find a person living in a house, evidently damp or wet, I feel bound, if he be not hopelessly ill, to urge his instant removal to a drier location. I do this on the same principle that I should direct a man, with intermittent fever, to remove from a so-called malarious district; as I should urge a flight from Charleston, S. C., by a man threatened with yellow fever during its prevalence in that city; or finally, as I should press for the instant removal of a typhoidal patient from the vicinity of a cess-pool. If you ask me why I do so, what cause *can* exist in a damp soil, productive of consumption, I simply point you to these previously given facts and inferences therefrom, and reply that we know no more what is the essential element or mode of procedure of this obscure cause of consumption, than we know of the causes of fever and ague, yellow or typhoid fever, above alluded to. If we wait until we understand the precise operation of causes before we take action, our action is, or may be, vain.

IX. — Apparent Exceptions, given by different Physicians, to the view of the subject presented in this Address.

The correspondents of one hundred and thirteen towns answered categorically and often monosyllabically in the negative, to the question as to the greater prevalence of consumption in one part, than elsewhere in the town. In other words, these practitioners have never seen in their town any particular locality, peculiarly liable to the prevalence of consumption. Thirty-nine of these answered doubtfully in the negative, or suggested some other reason than locality as the cause of its greater prevalence in one part of the town than another — *e. g.* the hereditary character of the affection in certain families, the peculiar trade, bad ventilation, a dusty atmosphere, &c. Two of them only give statistics — viz., Dr. Alden, of Randolph, and Dr. Cotting, of Roxbury. I refer elsewhere* for these data. I would, however, make the following criticism upon them.

There is a fatal omission in both, viz., that they give no means of comparing the number of deaths by consumption in the wet districts, either with the population or with the total deaths by all diseases. Now it is obvious, that unless we have one or the other of these latter data, we cannot make any assertion in the premises. For example: Dr. Cotting says there were only three deaths near the "mill-pond," and "but two on the ridge between the empty and full basin." But unless we know the relative population in these districts, or the total deaths, we are still in the dark in regard to the comparative rate of mortality from this cause. His own table, "Localities of the Deaths by Consumption," admits of doubt in regard to the conclusions he draws from it. For certainly, Dr. Cotting will allow that much more than two-thirds of the surface of the city of Roxbury cannot be called low. But only two-thirds of all the deaths in the city are found in the high localities, whereas, if consumption pre-

---

* Appendix F.

vailed everywhere alike, we ought to have many more than two-thirds.

It is plain, however, that we argue in vain, owing to the want of a necessary element of the evidence.

Again, it may be remarked, that as Roxbury is a somewhat densely built city, we may not be able to discover the influence of any telluric cause, as easily as in a township, more sparsely built upon, and extending over a larger space, of miles, perhaps, in extent.

"Every year," says Dr. Cotting, "brings accounts of some new and peculiarly favored locality, and every year brings also statistics, proving that any boasted exemption will not not bear the test of careful investigation. From the East Indies and the West, from isles of the ocean and those of the Mediterranean, from Western prairies and from Italian skies, we hear the same stories of the universal existence, prevalence and inexorable progress of pulmonary consumption." Upon this question I have simply to say, that such men, as Mühry in Germany, Lombard in Switzerland, Boudin in France, Coolidge in America, upon well-authenticated statistics, hold a totally opposite opinion.

Dr. Alden's data are subject to criticisms similar to those made on Dr. Cotting's. They afford no means of really comparing the number of deaths by consumption with the total deaths or population.

I do but justice, however, to Dr. A. in saying that he believes that a residence in a low damp spot is promotive of all diseases, consumption among the rest.

I have thus stated the opinion of those who differ from my estimate of the influence of dampness of the soil, as a cause of consumption.

I turn now to some important practical questions and suggestions, naturally arising from the subject.

Are there any Localities in New England which, from these Investigations, we should deem unfitted for the Residence of Consumptive Patients?

I believe that all towns, parts of towns, houses even that *rest on* damp, cold soils, are by that very fact peculiarly liable to the prevalence of consumption. I believe that similar locations *near* wet meadows, rivers, marshes, &c., though less subject to the law, are nevertheless, in a lesser degree, promoters of consumption in the families resident thereupon. Even hills, with a clayey subsoil retaining moisture, though not absolutely evil, are less good than a perfectly dry, porous soil, removed from any moisture. I suspect, moreover, that we ought to inquire more particularly than we have heretofore done, as to the exact condition of the cellar of a residence, whether it be damp or dry, even when the surroundings of the residence may seem perfectly good. All these statements I make, not on theory alone, but from actual experience, I think, of their truth, as learned from my professional practice during the past four or five years.

Again: on theoretical, but I believe just grounds, I have objected to allowing consumptive patients to reside in houses, *heavily and closely* shaded by trees and vines; because the rays of the sun being prevented from reaching such abodes, dampness and extra coolness are thereby promoted. I know of a house, which I should deem unfit for a consumptive to reside in. It is situated in New Hampshire, about fifty miles from Boston, on rather a low spot of ground. Its wooden sills rest, almost immediately, on the wet soil. Trees, thick and close, overshadow its roof, and woodbines cover its walls. When I visited it, one consumptive child was dying, and the sister was beginning to fail. I objected to the trees and vines, as tending, in that instance, to promote dampness and coolness, as above described.

Following out this idea, I have at times *thinned out* trees around a residence, where a family was growing up, and among which one had already shown signs of tubercular disease.

Looking at the subject from the opposite standpoint,

ARE THERE NOT PLACES WHICH, ACCORDING TO THESE INVESTIGATIONS, WILL TEND TO PREVENT PHTHISIS, OR AT LEAST, IN WHICH CONSUMPTION WILL PREVAIL MUCH LESS THAN ELSEWHERE, OR POSSIBLY NOT AT ALL?

I do not absolutely know a single spot in New England, where consumption can be said, by statistics, never to have occurred. In choosing a site for a dwelling-house, the great desideratum is to obtain, not a perfectly *arid* place, for no such spot could be inhabited by man, but it should be in a portion of the township which is neither so high as to be exposed to violent gusts of weather, nor so low that moisture will collect around it. Let it be on the side of a hill, or plain, open to the south, and, if possible, defended from the north and east, on a dry, porous soil, through which water freely percolates, and which, even after a rain, retains little moisture. Let the cellar be dry, in which no mould will collect. Such a situation, I believe, on theory (confirmed by my general experience), if it can be found in any town in New England, will be more favorable for the consumptive, and less likely to have consumption appear in it, than another spot, with a different exposure, and having a wet soil. So much for theory.

Places which Experience has taught me are Residences favorable for Consumptives.

There are two distinct classes of townships and localities, which I should place in this category. They are either inland towns, or islands eight or ten miles from the shore, and thereby being, in reality, under an oceanic climate. Doubtless, there are many more localities, besides those I shall name, scattered in almost all the inland portions of the New England States. These spots must be eventually discovered by the registration agents, or by the careful and conscientious investigations of resident physicians. I have had actual experience of the advantages of placing patients at Grantville, a district in the township of

Needham; also upon the drier portions of Sharon and of Canton, and at the Isles of Shoals. All these towns lie about ten or fifteen miles inland, while the islands are about the same distance from the coast. The former have the land; the latter, the oceanic climatic influences. The townships are remarkable for the dryness of their soil, and are generally somewhat elevated. In every one of them, I have had patients improve greatly, and some, whom I believe would have died in low coast, or wet inland spots, have recovered, or have speedily improved from serious symptoms. The patients have all described a decided and peculiar effect, as having been produced on their lungs by the atmosphere of these places, whereby they were enabled to breathe more easily.

The Isles of Shoals are off Portsmouth, New Hampshire. From the reports of physicians I have little doubt that Nantucket, Martha's Vineyard, and possibly Block Island, lying south of Massachusetts and Rhode Island, must be likewise useful.*

It may be objected, that in suggesting an island, I virtually ignore all my previous statements, in regard to the influence of moisture, as a cause of consumption. I answer, 1st—That it is evident that a small island, with an oceanic climate, may and probably would produce very different effects on a patient from those caused by a place on low and damp land. Hence the two places are evidently under wholly different influences. The two spots are not analo-

* I am also inclined to believe that Nahant and Winthrop, rocky promontories projecting from the coast, will prove favorable sites.

gous. But, 2d—In the places I have named, I, in reality, do not vary from the rule of dryness of the soil, for all of them are either mere rocks, rising out of the ocean, with no marshes near, or they are masses of sand, so to speak, and essentially dry of character. Hence they do, in reality, fall within the rule—only they have the oceanic atmosphere instead of the land atmosphere, encircling and covering them.

Whether this is really a correct explanation or not, I am certain that, in many cases of early phthisis, the tonic, clear, soft air of the Isles of Shoals, in summer, has been of immense service. Two patients spent the winter there. In one patient, a crackling throughout the whole of one breast disappeared, which I fear it would not have done, had the patient remained in Boston. The winds were violent, but the temperature was less severe than in corresponding places on the shore. These winds will, however, always prevent many from residing at the Shoals during the winter, unless, perchance, the inherent healthfulness of the situation, and the superb marine views, that one can enjoy there, should, in some future time, cause a Sanatarium to be erected, properly constructed to obviate, at least in part, these difficulties.*

* It is part of my medical faith, that, within fifty years, our community will occupy this and its kindred islands, as places peculiarly fitted for many of our citizens, who prefer to remain near home to seeking health further south. They will be in some measure, to New England, what the Isle of Wight is to Great Britain, although the beauties of the two places will be forever very different, and the climate of the Shoals less gracious than that of the mild, almost tropical, airs of Undercliff, or that of the islands of Nantucket, Martha's Vineyard, on our own shores, which experience some of the genial influences of the Gulf Stream.

General Summary of these Investigations, and of, what I deem, the logical Inferences the Public and the Profession should draw therefrom, with some Remarks on the Duties of the State, of the Public and of the Medical Profession, in relation to the Subject.

Commencing these investigations without any thought of ever arriving at these results, but simply with a hearty faith that every sincere student of God's laws on this planet will always find *more* than he can dare hope for, I have been led to, what I deem, one of the most important results of my professional studies.

By the examination of the State Registration Reports, all imperfect as they are; from the opinions of physicians, given in correspondence to me from one hundred and eighty-two towns in the Commonwealth; from the still more valuable statistics, afforded by some physicians in Massachusetts and her sister States; from the Army Reports; and finally from my own experience in practice, I have come to a firm belief in the following propositions:—

First. *Consumption is not equally distributed over New England.*

Second. *Its greater or less prevalence depends very much upon the characteristics of the soil on, or near which the patients affected with it have resided.*

Third. *Moisture of the soil is the only known characteristic that, so far as our present investigations have gone, is connected with the consumption breeding districts.*

FOURTH. *An attention to this law in the development of consumption in New England (now first, nearly, if not quite, proved to be true, by the analysis of the data which your courtesy has afforded me), I have found of great advantage in my professional practice.*

To the first three propositions, I have given you, I hope, sufficient evidence to command your close attention hereafter, in your various circuits of practice, even if they do not immediately gain your implicit belief. To the last proposition you, of course, will give just that amount of credence you think due to my judgment and my integrity.

But give me leave to say still further, that you have no right, I think, as honest men, to throw aside evidence, however trivial in certain respects it may seem, with an ill-suppressed sneer, or the simple remark that you, as individuals, cannot find any proof of the truth of my statements, in your own city or township. By so doing, you virtually declare that all the evidence given by your friends and neighboring physicians, throughout the State and adjacent States — quite equal probably to yourselves, in their opportunities and powers of observation, and from which evidence I have simply drawn out the essential truth —is of no worth whatever against your own individual opinion.

Allow me to press this view still further home upon your intellects and consciences, by a renewed appeal to the terrible mortality from consumption, already alluded to (p. 34), and my remarks thereupon. Let me, also, in this connection ask, if it be not possible that some of the cases of what is now evidently hereditary consumption, in certain families, may not be really the legitimate results of some ancestor's unfortunate place of residence. This may seem a peculiarly fanciful suggestion, but is by no means incredible. Although we cannot, at present, solve this and other important questions, naturally connected with the subject, I claim that the data, already given, ought, at least, to command the earnest attention of every member of this society.

If these things are so, what ought the State, the individual private citizen, and the Medical Profession, to do in the premises?

Let me say a few words on each division of this subject.

(*a*) The State has been and is now recreant to its duties, as a conservator of the public health, in not having, long ere this, carried out not only this but similar investigations upon all the diseases of New England. When I commenced my investigations, I arranged my questions with the sole purpose of comparing the results, obtained from my correspondents in different towns in regard to the hygiene of the towns, with the mortuary statistics of each, as given by the State Reports. I spent many precious hours examining the original records in the archives at the State House. But I finally gave up the attempt as utterly vain, as I found that they were, at that time, unreliable for particular towns, though, for the State at large, some general averages might be obtained. I hope, under the new law, better things are done. But I sincerely believe that very little of valuable information on the topographical distribution of disease will ever be accomplished, so long as the registration of vital statistics is left in the hands of men, non-professional, and who have no just appreciation of the difficulties or the value of such investigations. The State has spent its thousands for registration, and whatever good may have been done by the money thus spent, it is a lamentable fact, as has been stated by one writer, that if the Commonwealth wanted to know where would be the most healthy location for the site of a hospital, prison, or almshouse, it could not obtain the information from its own records ; and to-morrow, if the question were on the selection of a site for a normal school, it would be decided as much by the money power, as by hygienic laws. Such institutions should be perfectly situated, and able to carry out all hygienic laws. The normal school should not only teach these laws, to our future teachers, but the school, hospital and prison should be themselves models, in every respect, of obedience to those laws.

As much should be done by the legislature for public health, as is done by it for agriculture and education. Certainly, a Board of Health, composed of the ablest of the profession, and of others interested in vital statistics, is quite as important as Boards of Agriculture or of Education. Such a board could properly investigate every question of this kind, and if efficient, and armed, as it would be, with all the power of the State, it would gain data for the elucidation of any medical question, which no private individual could obtain.

(*b*) The public should correct its own views upon the whole subject of the planting of cities and villages. It should not allow speculators to run the risk of contaminating every family that may subsequently colonize a spot, the best fitted, perhaps, for the promotion of consumption. Now, the track of the railway, or the wit or reckless energy of the owner of some swamp, may be the sole reason for erecting a station house, and thereby promoting the early erection of dwelling-houses near by, on localities totally unfit for human habitations. I know of, at least, two villages thus built, in total contravention of this law of consumption. To one I am called, I think, oftener for cases of consumption than to any of its neighboring townships.*

Such villages might probably be much improved, if not made perfectly healthy locations, by thorough *under-drainage.* The public, however, is not aware of the value of such drainage. It may be that the suggestion will seem an infringement on private rights, but I am inclined to think that this whole matter of the location of cities ought to be somewhat more under the control of law, than it is at present. No man or body of men has a right to set up a nuisance. If a man has not wisdom or generosity enough to forbear inviting the public to live in locations that are, in themselves, nuisances of the worst kind, then public law ought to restrain

---

* This village was commenced only a few years ago, and the greater part of the land directly adjacent to it can be put under water at any time, according to the caprice of a mill-dam corporation, which commands the village stream. Can anything be more absurd?

11

him, as it would restrain him from doing any other obviously evil thing to the community.

(*c*) What can private individuals do in this matter? Let every one, if possible, keep himself and family away from any permanent residence in a house whose foundations are constantly surrounded by the exhalations from a damp soil of meadow or marsh, or even hill, that is full of springs, and which consequently keep the cellar of the habitation moist and cold. If perchance ignorantly he has erred, and finds a puny set of children growing up around him, in a house thus situated, let him take warning and flee from it, before it be too late. This is no fancy sketch. Our statistics prove the possibility of a childless old age, in consequence of too long a residence in such a place.

What should the Profession do, in reference to this Subject?

Finally, Gentlemen, what ought the Profession —what ought we, individually, to do in our respective localities, and as members of a Profession which ought to be the proper guardian of the Public Health?

Persuade the State to establish a Board of Health.

We are bound, as already stated, as a body, not to let the Legislature have peace from our annual petitions, until a system of investigations, similar to, though more thorough than that which I have presented in this Address, shall be made on the topographical distribution of all diseases, by an able and appropriately elected State Board of Health. I may seem unduly earnest, but it appears to me that our Society could not do a better act, one that will eventually be of more service, not only to the inhabitants of this State, but, by its example also, to other States, than by united and persistent effort to induce the State authorities to establish a State Board of Health, by whose agencies all these great questions, now utterly ignored, may be investigated. Under such a Board, and with such objects, vital statistics would become a matter of much more personal interest than it is at present.

Endeavor to use this Law in a Prophylactic point of view.

But the results at which we have already arrived, even in these investigations, ought to come home, I think, to the judgment and consciences of every member of the Society, in his daily walk of practice. There are, I doubt not, in every township, one or more families, that are slowly being undermined in health; members of them are either preparing to fall victims to consumption, or, if perchance they escape with puny constitutions, their offspring may be essentially cachectic and tuberculous, thus entailing misery upon generations yet unborn. And all this is being done, as I fear, in pure ignorance of one of the great primal laws of the development of consumption in New England. You will readily imagine what I, at least, claim, that it would be the duty of every member of this Society to do in a like case. He should declare, in terms not to be misunderstood, that as parents who go on year after year, living in such an abode and having children born unto them, are virtually the makers, so they are by as certain, though perchance slower process, the slayers of their race! This doubtless seems severe; and in avowing such an opinion, in any particular case, you may meet not only all the violent opposition arising from ignorance of Nature's law, but also the more powerful influence of pecuniary interest—of affection, perhaps, for a venerated homestead. Parents may perhaps have entered the abode after confirmed adult life. They may have lived many years on the spot. Every birth has added a new charm, and a new and sweeter association to it. Their own healths have not been *materially* influenced. They will argue, as they may think, very philosophically, when saying, "We have lived here twenty years, and *we* have not died of consumption. How, then, can it be the abode that produces the disease in our children?" This is also, Gentlemen, no fancy argument. Almost the precise words have been used to me. In vain, perhaps, will you say that the argument wholly falls to the ground, because the two cases are not alike; the tender and sensitive nature of childhood being much more susceptible to all external impressions, than is the hardened nature of adult life.

The reasons why our argument fails of its object, and the parents still cling to their fatal abode, may be various, but one of the most cogent is the fact that neither public opinion nor the opinion of physicians has ever taken the ground I now assume.

To that point I would endeavor to bring you, and, through you, the public at large.

Use the Law in the Treatment of individual Cases of Disease.

But we shall all be thrown more closely in contact with the operation of the law of soil-moisture, when we come to the treatment of individual cases. I would draw your attention to a few of them.

We may meet with a patient suffering under what is sometimes inaptly called the "pretubercular condition," where there is a general disturbance of the system—a *good-for-nothingness*—a languor, in fact, of body and soul, in the performance of their functions, perhaps a slight dyspepsia, some emaciation and debility—a little cough, but without *physical* signs of pulmonary disease. If such a patient have been residing under the circumstances named in this Address, as promotive of consumption, *it will be our first duty to urge him to leave the spot.* If he be living in the northern rooms of the house, where no sun can reach him, especially if the rooms have a damp, bleak exposure, he should remove to one which is bathed with the warm rays of noon. I have, in two cases of debility analogous to that described, seen great and immediate benefits result. One patient delighted in sitting hour after hour with the full force of the sun lying upon her whole form below the head. She seemed to imbibe strength and life from this, to her, novel sun-bath.

Do we not all of us, even while in perfect health, unconsciously recognize by our lungs, if in no other way, the oppressiveness of a room which, during any period of the year, has been, for any reason, shut from the sun's rays, even for a single day? We do not breathe as easily, and the mind becomes sluggish in such a place. How much more, then, should we guard those whose lungs are threatened with disease, from this extra suffering! Yet how utterly regardless is this community of all consideration of the influence of sun-light on health, though very earnest, perhaps, when the question arises of preserving the color of a fine painting or the brilliant hues of an expensive carpet! I write not poetry, but simple fact, when I say that on these occasions, sometimes, in our gross ignorance of God's laws, we risk blanching the human "face divine," in our eager desire to preserve a mere work of art or an expensive luxury. Pardon this apparent digression from the main current of our investigations, to which I now return.

Still more should a removal be urged if any, even the most trivial, of physical signs of pulmonary disease be found. A short distance, even of half or quarter of a mile, may do much good; but I should prefer to have such a patient remove at once to one of the places already known, or which may hereafter be found to be drier and more favorable for him. It has been stated that, in my zeal for retaining our patients in Massachusetts, I oppose entirely their removal to the more southern climates of Florida, Cuba, and of Europe. Nothing could be further from the truth; but where one is able to travel for health, thousands are fastened by the iron grasp of necessity to their native soil, and to but a very small space of even that. They cannot leave their own village. This law offers up some chance for even these.

Use it so as to cut off one of the main Causes of Consumption in New England.

But the most important result, that I hope will arise from these investigations, is on the future *prevention,* rather than the cure of phthisis in Massachusetts. We have, in a previous portion of the Address, seen that, in some townships, twice or thrice as many die in the wet as in the dry districts. If this be so, and if an analogous state of things exists generally in Massachusetts, we must so indoctrinate our people that all wet spots shall be avoided as places of residence. No villages should be allowed to be planted on wet meadows or such like places, however much cupidity or convenience to railways may tend to induce capitalists to place them there. I am well aware of the evil influence such an opinion would have upon many public and private residences, now or hereafter to be occupied, while it would justly raise others in the estimation of the people. If, however, consumption can be, in the least, checked by such doctrines, it is our duty to proclaim them, in spite of all considerations of a pecuniary nature. If we once bring the public to this belief, we shall cut off, if not the "tap-root," at least one of the principal roots of consumptive tendencies in New England.

In conclusion, Gentlemen, let me say, that, I am sure, you will not doubt that I have full confidence in the truth of every assertion I have presented to you; and let me beg each one of you, in terms similar to those I used in commencing my Address, to ponder well what I have presented, and to bring it all to the test of your unbiassed daily experience. If the law I have announced be founded in Nature, it will stand, in spite of your individual opposition. If, perchance, I have unwittingly led myself and others towards error, by your efforts shall I, and many more who now believe as I do, be sooner brought back to Truth.

APPENDIX.

B.*

In June, 1854, at the request of the Massachusetts Medical Society, I undertoook to report on the following question:—

"Pulmonary Consumption: its relative mortality in different regions of the State; and the real or apparent connection of this mortality with the physical character of the different regions, and with the social and industrial condition of the inhabitants."

Accordingly, I issued the following series of questions, on three separate occasions, viz., January and March, 1854, and February 28, 1858.

At the last issue, I appended the note, dated February 23, 1858.

Returns from all the townships in Massachusetts (325) were made. Upon 183 of them, the Medical Opinion, alluded to in the Address, is based.

This Medical Opinion has been derived in the following manner. If a correspondent, in answer to the circular given below, stated, or occasionally though briefly gave statistics to prove, that consumption was rife throughout a township, I have examined his answers to the other questions of the Circular, especially those to Nos. 1, 2, 3, 10, 11, 12, 13, 15. I have thus endeavored to decide the chief characteristics of the townships, in regard to the relative amount of moisture or dryness found in each. Similar examinations were made in regard to special localities, or houses in which consumption was said or known to have prevailed. And so on, with all the five classes of townships named in Table II. (p. 23).

The questions in my Circular were as follows:—

Name of Township, and its population.

1. Height above sea level?
2. Distance from sea?
3. Is sea breeze felt there?
4. What winds most troublesome to consumptive patients?
5. What winds—North, East, South or West—most prevalent?
6. Is town liable to sudden changes from heat to cold?
7. Is town liable to sudden changes from dryness to moisture?
8. Is any part of town peculiarly liable to the prevalence of Consumption?
9. If so, what, if any, are the peculiarities of the spot?

---

* For "A—Memorial," referred to in the Address, see "Obituaries," following the Appendix.

10. What is the atmosphere generally (cool? warm? dry? damp? foggy? &c.)?
11. What is the position of town (exposed? sheltered? warm? cold? &c.)?
12. Annual amount of rain (great? medium? small?)?
13. Annual amount of snow (" " ")?
14. Employments of citizens (farming? fishing? factories? trading? &c.)?
15. Soil (geological structure? rivers? ponds? bay? meadows? marshes? hills? valleys? &c.)?
16. Cultivation (very rich? good? medium? poor?)?
17. Social condition (rich? medium? poor? buildings? &c.)?

February 23, 1858.

Dear Sir,—Above is a copy of the Circular which has been circulated in Massachusetts. You will observe that some of the questions may be answered by simply underscoring certain words. Of course, I should like as much detail as you may be able or willing to give. Monosyllabic (at least) returns to these have been received from every town in Massachusetts, and from a few towns in the neighboring States of Vermont, New Hampshire, Maine and Rhode Island. What I especially want, however, now, are actual statistics of the prevalence of Consumption in the various portions of New England. For this purpose, several persons have given me, from their own knowledge, or from the information of others, the following facts, accompanied at times by a map (rough, perhaps, but very valuable) of the town, representing the districts, and marking their peculiarities of soil and climate generally. The facts I wish for, are as follows:—

Population of town.
Population (at least approximatively) of each district.
Number of deaths by *all* diseases in each district.
Number of deaths by consumption in each district.

Likewise, a brief answer to all the questions that can be readily answered in the above Circular. Respectfully yours,

HENRY I. BOWDITCH.

The following are the names of the various townships and resident correspondents, from whom I have received the data on which the preceding Address is founded. It is due to them that I thus publicly thank them for their extreme courtesy, and valuable information, obtained, at times, by them with much labor.

Abington,	Dr. A. P. Chase
Acton,	H. Cowdrey A. H. Cowdrey
Adams,	N. S. Babbitt
Alford,	M. R. Van Deusen
Amesbury,	Thos. Sparhawk
Amherst,	B. F. Smith
Andover,	
Ashby,	Alfred Hitchcock
Ashburnham,	Alfred Miller
Ashfield,	C. L. Knowlton
Ashland,	J. C. Harris
Athol,	George Hoyt George Field
Attleboro',	Thaddeus Phelps
Auburn,	J. E. Hathaway Daniel Green
Barnstable,	H. E. M'Collum
Barre,	Dr. J. M. Bates
Becket,	W. O. Bell
Bedford,	A. B. Adams
Belchertown,	H. Thomson
Bellingham,	L. L. Scammell
Berkley,	Wm. Dickinson
Berlin,	
Bernardston,	John Brooks
Beverly,	Augustus Torrey Charles Haddock
Billerica,	Augustus Mason
Blackstone,	Abel Wilder
Blandford,	Silas P. Wright
Bolton,	Dr. W. H. Bigelow
Boston,	Mr. N. A. Appollonio
Boxboro',	C. Hartwell Cowdrey
Boxford,	W. S. Coggin

Boylston,	Dr. John Andrews
Bradford,	George Cogswell
Braintree,	Noah Torrey
Brewster,	S. H. Gould
Bridgewater,	Calvin B. Pratt
	A. T. Lowe
Brighton,	I. G. Braman
Brimfield,	A. Lincoln
Brookfield,	J. A. Penniman
Brookline,	Charles Wild
Buckland,	J. Trow
Burlington,	Rev. Samuel Sewall
Byfield,	Dr. Martin Root
Cambridge	M. Wyman
Cambridgeport	W. W. Wellington
Canton,	C. S. Taft
Carlisle,	Austin Marsh
Carver,	H. T. Erland
Charlemont,	M. F. Potter
Charlestown,	A. R. Thompson
Charlton,	C. M. Fay
	Isaac Porter
Chatham,	E. W. Carpenter
Chelmsford,	N. B. Edwards
Cheshire,	L. L. Cole
Chester,	Mr. E. D. Cooke
	E. L. Hill
	H. S. Lucas
Chesterfield,	Dr. A. M. Smith
Chicopee,	P. L. B. Stickney
Chilmark,	R. R. Jones
Clarksburg,	N. S. Babbitt
Clinton,	G. W. Burdett
Cohasset,	Joseph Osgood
	C. C. Tower
Coleraine,	A. C. Deane
Concord,	H. A. Barrett
Conway,	E. D. Hamilton
Cummington,	Mr. Swain
Dalton,	Dr. Henry Ferre
Dana,	Albert Amsden
Danvers,	Eben Hunt
Dartmouth,	W. B. Mason
Dedham,	J. Stimson
Deerfield,	G. F. Gale
Dennis,	C. M. Hurlbert
Dighton,	Wm. Dickinson
Dorchester,	Edward Jarvis
	John P. Spooner
	E. D. Miller
Douglass,	J. E. Sinnell
Dover,	Rev. Ralph Sanger
Dracut,	Dr. Henry Richardson
Dudley,	S. F. Lindsey
Dunstable,	A. P. Pierce
Duxbury,	Mr. Seth Sprague
	Dr. James Wilde

E. Bridgewater,	Dr. Samuel Orr
E. Cambridge,	Moses Clark
Easthampton,	Atherton Clark
Eastham,	John Phillips
Easton,	John H. Gushee
	Caleb Swan
Edgarton,	J. H. Lucas
Egremont,	J. M. Bassett
Enfield,	E. H. Rockwood
	J. W. Winslow
Erving,	Edward Barton
Essex,	Josiah Lamson
Fairhaven,	George Atwood
	Paul Spooner
Fall River,	R. T. Davis
Falmouth,	Aaron Cornish
Fitchburg,	T. R. Boutelle
	L. Pillsbury
Florida,	N. S. Babbitt
Foxboro',	J. G. S. Hitchcock
Framingham,	S. Whitney
Franklin,	L. L. Scammell
Freetown,	Thos. G. Nichols
Gardner,	J. H. Greenwood
Georgetown,	George Moody
Gill,	J. Lyons
Gloucester,	H. E. Davidson
	J. F. Dyer
Goshen,	Daniel Pierce
Grafton,	D. Pierce
Granby,	C. N. Chamberlain
Granville,	Vincent Holcomb
Grt. Barrington,	N. B. Pickett
Greenfield,	James Deane
Greenwich,	C. E. Davis
Groton,	Joshua Green
Groveland,	Jeremiah Spofford
Hadley,	Franklin Bonney
Halifax,	Edwin Inglee
Hamilton,	D. S. Allen
Hancock,	Frank A. Cady
Hanover,	B. Whitwell
Hanson,	Bowen Barker
Hardwick,	Almon M. Orcutt
	J. P. Lynde
Harwich,	Franklin Dodge
Harvard,	E. A. Holman
Hatfield,	T. S. Knight
Haverhill,	Kendall Flint
Hawley,	Henry Seymour
Heath,	Cyrus Temple
Hingham,	R. T. P. Fiske
Hinsdale,	B. F. Kittredge
Holden,	A. D. Smith
Holland,	David B. Dean
Holliston,	E. G. Plympton
Hopkinton,	J. Pratt

Holyoke,	Dr. A. B. Clark
Hubbardston,	Moses Phelps
Hull,	Mr. Samuel Loring
Ipswich,	Dr. C. H. Brown
Kingston,	P. L. Nichols
Lakeville,	Isaac Sampson
Lancaster,	J. L. S. Thompson
Lanesboro',	Mr. G. R. Rockwell
Lawrence,	Dr. Seneca Sargent
Lee,	Coridon Guiteau
Leicester,	Edward Flint
Lenox,	M. Sabin
Leominster,	C. C. Field
Leverett,	David Pierce
Lexington,	Howland Holmes
Leyden,	E. Haynes
Lincoln,	H. C. Chapin
Littleton,	J. G. Eliot
Longmeadow,	George Hooker
Lowell,	J. C. Dalton
Ludlow,	W. B. Alden
Lunenburg,	D. Manning
Lynn,	James M. Nye
Lynnfield,	John Perkins, Jr.
Malden,	Nathan French
Manchester,	L. B. Farrar
Mansfield,	W. F. Perry
Marblehead,	C. Blaisdell
Marion,	W. N. Ellis
Marlboro',	E. H. Barnes
Marshfield,	Henry Blanchard
Marshpee,	Mr. Chas. Marston
Mason,	Dr. W. N. Ellis
Medfield,	John S. Galloup
Medford,	C. V. Bemis
	Milton Fuller
Medway,	S. Salisbury
	Ira Perry
Melrose,	Moses Parker
Mendon,	J. G. Metcalf
Methuen,	J. M. Grosvenor
Middleboro',	J. Perkins
Middlefield,	S. F. Root
Middleton,	E. S. Phelps
Milford,	Francis Leland
Millbury,	Henry G. Davis
Milton,	Jonathan Ware
Monson,	Alvan Smith
Montague,	David Bradford
Monterey,	Alvan H. Turner
Montgomery,	S. Shurtleff
Mt. Washington	H. W. Lamson
Munroe,	H. Gould, of Rowe
Nantucket,	E. P. Fearing
Natick,	Ira Russell
Needham,	Edward Warren

New Ashford,	Leland White
Newbury,	Dr. Martin Root
Newburyport,	H. C. Perkins
New Bedford,	W. A. Gordon
	Lyman Bartlett
New Braintree,	A. A. Kendall
New Marlboro',	J. P. Perkins
New Salem,	Robert Andrews
Newton Centre,	W. H. Thayer
Newton U. Falls	Edward Warren
Northampton	E. E. Denniston
N. Bridgewater,	Horatio Bryant
	A. K. Borden
N. Brookfield,	J. Porter, Jr.
Northboro',	Joseph Allen
	C. W. Barnes
Northbridge,	R. R. Clarke
Northfield,	Elijah Stratton
Norton,	W. Dickinson
Norwich,	T. K. De Wolf
Oakham,	S. P. Martin
Orange,	Ed. Barton
Orleans,	Benj. F. Seabury
Otis,	M. Webb
Oxford,	Jonathan Nichols
Palmer,	Jason B. Thomas
Pawtucket,	B. Carpenter
Paxton,	E. M. Wheeler
Pelham,	A. G. Craig
Pembroke,	Francis Collamore
Pepperell,	N. Cutter
	Chas. E. Parker
Peru,	Frank. A. Cady
Petersham,	Sam'l Taylor
Phillipston,	Jason Goulding
Pittsfield,	Frank. A. Cady
Plainfield,	Sam'l Shaw
Plymouth,	Le Baron Russell
Plympton,	J. T. Hammond
Prescott,	Daniel Lowell
Princeton,	W. N. Boylston
Provincetown,	John L. Lothrop
Quincy,	Eben'r Woodward
Randolph,	Eben'r Alden
Randolph, E.	T. E. Wood
Raynham,	Elisha Hayward
Reading,	H. P. Wakefield
Reading, N.	" "
Reading, S.	J. D. Mansfield
Rehoboth,	M. R. Randall
Richmond,	
Rochester,	Joseph Haskell
	W. E. Sparrow
Rockport,	Benj. Haskell
Rowe,	Humphrey Gould
Rowley,	Richard Herbert

Roxbury,	Dr. B. E. Cotting
Royalston,	Isaac P. Willis
Russell,	S. Shurtleff
Rutland,	B. H. Tripp
Salem,	G. Choate
Salisbury,	Benj. Sawyer
Sandisfield,	Erastus Beach
Sandwich,	John Bachelder Henry Russell
Saugus,	Sam'l Hawks
Savoy,	A. M. Bowker
Scituate,	Francis Thomas
" *S.*	Rev. Caleb Stetson
Seekonk,	Dr. Johnson Gardner
Sharon,	A. D. Bacon
Sheffield,	Oliver Peck
Shelburne,	Chas. M. Duncan
Sherborn,	A. C. Blanchard
Shirley,	James O. Parker
Shrewsbury,	Adolph. Brigham
Shutesbury,	Lewis S. Bemis
Somerset,	John B. Chase
Somerville,	Luther V. Bell
Southampton,	Artemas Bell
Southboro,'	Mr. Joseph Burnett
Southbridge,	Dr. S. C. Hartwell
South Hadley,	Ed. G. Ufford
Southwick,	J. W. Rockwell
Spencer,	Jonas Guilford
Springfield,	Alfred Lambert
Sterling,	Thos. H. Gage
Stockbridge,	Mr. E. H. Owen
Stoneham,	Dr. W. F. Stevens
Stoughton,	Simeon Tucker J. B. Walker
Stowe,	Hermon Chandler
Sturbridge,	Calvin P. Fiske
Sudbury,	L. Goodenough
Sunderland,	Nath'l G. Trow
Sutton,	William Terry
Swansea	J. L. Wellington
Taunton,	Wm. Dickinson
Templeton,	J. W. D. Osgood
Tewksbury,	Jonathan Brown
Tisbury,	R. K. Jones
Tolland,	F. D. Austin
Topsfield,	R. A. Merriam
Townsend,	E. Leigh
Truro,	J. H. Davis
Tyngsboro',	Aug. F. Pierce
Tyringham,	Alvan H. Turner

Upton,	Dr. H. Carpenter
Uxbridge,	Jas. W. Robbins
Wales,	Jno. Smith
Walpole,	Eben. Stone
Waltham,	H. Adams
Ware,	E. C. Richardson
Wareham,	P. F. Doggett
Warren,	Nelson Carpenter
Warwick,	Amos Taylor
Washington,	
Watertown,	Hiram Hosmer
Wayland,	Jacob Ulman
Webster,	Charles Negus
Wellfleet,	Solomon A. Rich
Wendell,	L. Cooke
Wenham,	Nathan Jones
Westboro',	Benj Pond
West Boylston,	Ephraim Lovell
W. Bridgewater,	Daniel Chaplin
W. Brookfield,	Wm. Curtis
W. Cambridge	Jos. Underwood
W. Stockbridge,	R. H. Comstock
Westfield,	J. Abbott
Westford,	Benj. Osgood
Westhampton,	H. H. Orcutt
Westminster,	Wm. L. Lincoln
W. Newbury,	John Appleton
Weston,	Otis E. Hunt
Westport,	B. B. Sisson
W. Roxbury,	Geo. Faulkner
W. Springfield,	Reuben Champion
Weymouth, N.	Noah Fifield
Whately,	Myron Harwood C. Bardwell, 2d
Wilbraham,	Jesse W. Price
Williamsburg,	T. Meekins Washington Shaw
Williamstown,	Henry L. Sabin S. Duncan
Wilmington,	B. Cutter
Winchendon,	Alvah Godding
Winchester,	A. Chapin
Windsor,	W. Richards
Winthrop,	P. M. Crane
Woburn,	Aug. Plympton B. Cutter
Worcester,	Wm. Workman
Worthington,	A. M. Smith
Wrentham,	D. L. Gibbens
Yarmouth,	George Shove

Correspondents in Maine.

Bethel,	Dr. John Grover
Dixmont,	A. Johnson
Kennebunk,	—— Trafton
Saccarappa,	Dr. Wm. Marrett
Saco,	J. L. Allen

Correspondents in New Hampshire.

Atkinson,	Dr. Isaac B. Hovey	*Farmington,*	Dr. C. L. Hartwell Charles Tuttle
Hampton,	C. H. Sanborn	*Greenland,*	G. C. Clough
Hampton Falls,	" "		
Newport,	S. E. Richardson		

Correspondents in Rhode Island.

Bristol and Warren, Drs. J. James Ellis and Charles W. Parsons.

D.

The following are the facts referred to in the Address. Dr. Ira Perry says: "Black Swamp is blamed for fevers, consumption, &c. In it, water is stagnant, in some parts most of the year. People around, however, live to a good old age. There is one spot on which there are three houses (the only ones except one new one), where, within twenty-five years, fourteen persons have died of consumption, confined to four families, a quarter of a mile apart. This spot is low, springy land on the north, and Charles River on the south, close by. The north-east winds drive directly over this swamp upon the houses."

In a subsequent letter, Dr. P. suggests, that perhaps the hereditary nature of the disease may have had effect.

Dr. Garratt, formerly of Hanover, now of Boston, informs me of a house in Pembroke, in which, he thought, before he knew of my views, that consumption commenced in a family, having no tendency to phthisis, in consequence of the presence of moisture and coldness. It is situated on a hill, and exposed to the full force of north and east winds from over the Marshfield flats, and through a valley, overflowed each spring and autumn. These winds, of course, come laden with moisture. But besides this, the house had behind it, and close upon it, a pool of water, about twenty feet square, into which all the refuse of the house and barn was conveyed, thus forming a festering mass of corruption, in addition to the moisture. Effluvia from this continually filled the house. Two of the children died of phthisis, and a third began to falter. The patient was removed from the spot, and the pool dried up at the earnest solicitation of Dr. G. After removal from the place, the family improved in health. Some may deem the filth more prominent, as a cause of the disease in this instance, than the moisture of the soil. Dr. G., however, who saw the place, believed that the constantly wet soil, immediately adjacent to the house, was the chief cause.

Dr. Brown, of Tewksbury, says the house where most cases of consumption have occurred, is "an old, ill-repaired and dilapidated house, standing about fifty rods from Shawshan River, on rather moist land, and in the shade of a very large willow tree."

Dr. Bartlett, of New Bedford (page 42), mentions a family in a town in the western part of the State, in which both parents and four out of five children died of consumption. This house is terribly situated, if we have any belief in the effect of moisture in producing consumption. Without this belief, we should say it was a pleasant summer residence. A mill-pond is directly behind it. It is in the depth of a mountain valley, and covered wholly from the sun by lofty and large outspreading shade trees. Heavy fogs rest often on this dwelling when the adjacent hills are free.

Dr. Bartlett also thinks that " nearly every one of both families died of consumption in two houses very near the last-named, and similarly bathed with moisture and covered with shade trees."

F.

Dr. Alden's statistics (p. 66), so far as they bear upon our immediate question, are as follows : —

Under date of February 17, 1854—out of 70 undoubted cases of well-known tubercular consumption, from 1820 to 1845, and excluding all either of a doubtful character or of which he says he has " no personal knowledge," and all being in American families—

18	occupied	elevated	situations.
39	"	medium	"
13	"	low	"

Subsequently I wrote to ask more particularly about the influence of moisture, it being evident that mere relative height does not show anything, in reality, about the amount of *moisture* of the soil in that same part. His answer is as follows :—

" In reply to your inquiry whether moisture or a residence near swamps or springy soil, or rivers or ponds, have been at all connected with the reported deaths, I answer "No," so far as my inquiries have extended. To enable you to appreciate the value of this answer, it will be necessary for me to say that the Blue Hill ridge is situated north of us, running in an easterly direction from the north-west corner of Randolph. Immediately south of this ridge is a chain of ponds, beginning westerly. (Dr. A. names six.) From these, there is a gentle ascent southerly, until, at a distance of from three to six miles, the height is reached which divides Massachusetts from Narragansett Bay. On this slope Randolph is situated, divided into East and West Randolph by a valley, running north and south, fifty feet or more lower than the grounds east and west, through which a small stream runs, originating in the swamps and meadows near the height of land, and receiving accessions from the ponds. * * The two principal streets of the town run parallel with the river, and at an average distance of one mile from it, and the great body of the inhabitants occupy sites, comparatively elevated. With these explanations, you will readily understand how it happened that, of the reported cases of phthisis, only thirteen had their residence near swamps or in damp situations."

It is evident, as remarked in the Address, that until we know the relative population on the parts alluded to, we cannot decide the question of the greater or less prevalence of consumption in them.

Dr. A. concludes his letter by saying, that his opinion is that the coldness and moisture of the low parts would "be adapted to work mischief on the organs of respiration, and if the population of such districts were equally dense with those which are more elevated, I have no doubt such a result would be apparent."

Dr. Cotting's arguments against the views taken in the Address (page 66), are contained in an elaborately prepared discourse, delivered before the Norfolk District Medical Society.* It is an answer to a circular, similar to my own, sent to the members by the Secretary, Dr. Jarvis. In order to show exactly what Dr. C.'s opinions are, I quote the following :—

III. — *Is it [Consumption] more prevalent along Water-Courses or near to Mill-Ponds that are alternately raised and drained off?*

We have been at some considerable pains-taking to mark, on a plan of the city, the localities of the deaths from consumption for the last four years; and have thus with tolerable accuracy indicated as many as could be ascertained, or 208 out of 257, the whole number.

By reference to this plan, it appears that along the only fresh-water *mill-pond* (that near Lowell Street), which is alternately raised and drained off, and where is often left exposed a large muddy surface, and on whose margins, with those of its inlet, are the principal low grounds bordering on fresh water, there have been but *three* deaths from consumption during the past four years; and these, so far as can be ascertained, originating clearly from causes not connected with the locality. Along the ridge of land between the full and empty basins of salt water of the "Boston Mill Company," in that part within the limits of Roxbury, but *two* deaths from consumption have been recorded during the same time.

IV. — *Has any Effect been observed of any other kind of Locality?*

On the borders of the marsh land, and the ridges immediately adjoining, there have been many deaths; but in these localities the population is most dense and of the most destitute classes. And even here the native population and the best and most comfortably housed of the foreigners seem to be as exempt from consumption as in other localities.

In such neighborhoods, from the comparative cheapness of land, the new emigrants erect their miserable tenements, and fill them to overflowing with such as either desire or are able to procure no better abodes. Crowded apartments (sometimes ten or a dozen persons, frequently half that number occupying for all purposes a room, say fifteen feet square); filthiness to an incredible degree in person and raiment; coarse and ill-cooked food, eaten in ravenous haste; intolerably oppressive and offensive atmospheres; excessive use of tobacco, and perhaps other bad habits; all these are prevalent among the denizens of such places, and are in a common-sense view of

---

* Statistics of Consumption in Roxbury. Read before the Norfolk District Medical Society of Massachusetts, at the Annual Meeting, May 17, 1854. By B. E. Cotting, M.D. Printed by vote of the Society.

the matter as likely to be productive of disease, even the disease in question, as the resting of their habitations on low and damp foundations.*

This view seems to be sustained in the following tables, constructed for the purpose of throwing some light on these points.

Descent of those dead from all Diseases.

Year.	Roxbury born.	Other Americans.	Foreign Immigrants.	Total.
1850—51	145	93	95	333
1851—52	139	115	121	375
1852—53	118	96	83	297
1853—54	161	96	91	348

Descent of those dead from Consumption.

Year.	Roxbury born.	Other Americans.	Foreign Immigrants.	Total.
1850—51	11	21	27	59
1851—52	12	29	34	73
1852—53	10	25	37	74
1853—54	6	21	24	51

According to the State Census, taken in 1850, the proportion of Americans to foreigners and children of foreign parents, in the five lower wards, now constituting the city of Roxbury, was as follows:

	Americans.	Children of Foreign Parents.	Foreigners.	Total.
	8347	1921	4882	15150

---

* Since the above went to press, through the kindness of Drs. Harris and Weld, of Jamaica Plain, I have been furnished with a transcript from the Church Records of sixty-seven cases of death from consumption, which occurred in that Parish (embracing the middle third part of the area of the original city of Roxbury), from Feb. 7, 1793, to Jan. 7, 1847—a period of fifty-four years. These cases I have carefully examined and classed as follows.

Deaths from Consumption at Jamaica Plain, from 1793 *to* 1847.

High and dry Ground.	High near Low Ground.	Low Ground.	Salt Marsh.	Came in last Stages.	Location not known.	Total.
26	12	4	1	10	14	67

Of these cases, 26 occurred on high and dry ground; 12 on high land, within an eighth or a quarter of a mile of a meadow, brook or pond; 4 on low grounds; 1 near a narrow strip of salt marsh which touches the parish at one of its corners; 10 came into the place in the last stages of the disease; and the locations of 14 are not stated, and are not now known. Ten of the dead are spoken of in the records, as having been of consumptive families; of which 4 were on high ground, 2 near low, 2 on low, and 2 on locations not stated.

[In not stating the number of the inhabitants or the total number of deaths in each district, these statistics prove really nothing for or against the doctrines of the Address.—H. I. B.]

Thus it is evident that while the proportion of immigrant foreigners to Americans and the children born here of foreign parents, is as 48 to 102, or less than one third, and while the deaths from all causes to the immigrants amount to only one in three or four of the whole number; nearly, and in some instances, quite half of all the deaths from consumption occur amongst the immigrants.

Furthermore, it may be seen by the following table, that the number of those who died from consumption, and who were known to have dwelt on low, wet, or made lands, where many of the immigrant population reside, amount to 78 out of 257, or a little less than one third—while those who died of consumption on high and dry lands, amount to 170, or two thirds of the whole number.

Localities of the Deaths from Consumption.

Year.	High.	Low.	Not known.	Total.
1850—51	33	11	15	59
1851—52	31	25	17	73
1852—53	42	23	9	74
1853—54	24	19	8	51
1850—1854	170	78	49	257

Dr. Cotting closes his Address in the following words:

"We are aware that to draw general conclusions from observations over limited portions of space and time, as well as from other partial premises, is a very common error. We shall therefore only venture to express the opinion that the causes of consumption are infinitely various, that the disease may arise wherever any vice exists in the individual system, originating from ancestry, external circumstances, or internal derangements—from any cause, in short, which depresses the system below a natural, healthy or normal standard, despite of, or in conjunction with, the influences emanating from the locality. The peculiar condition of the soil beneath, or the air above, the prevalence of vapors, or the absence of them, may seem at one time greatly to influence the disease; but in another and different period they appear to have no effect whatever upon it. No place which is now exempt, or for a few years past has been comparatively free from this disease, can boast of its exemption with any certainty that the boast, even as it passes the lips, may not prove empty and in vain.

"In the present state of our knowledge, consumption appears to be a method designed to remove those whose mortal bodies have, from whatever cause, fallen below the normal condition: and, as such, however much it may be ameliorated, is not likely ever to be extinguished while the same nature is continued to the human race."

In the Address, I have made the remarks I deemed necessary on the views held by Dr. Cotting. I have felt it to be my duty to present all the facts I could obtain, in opposition to my views on this very important question in the Etiology of consumption in Massachusetts.

Upon this conclusion, to which Dr. Cotting arrives, I would simply remark that such a belief as this, if applied generally in the investigation of all diseases, would forever check improvement in medical art—all hopes of ever relieving poor human nature of any of the various ills to which it is liable. Dr. Cotting would undoubtedly shrink from such a conclusion. But what right, *a priori*, has Dr. Cotting to say that consumption is selected, *par excellence*, as the favorite means used by Almighty Power for sweeping off the refuse of mankind, and is therefore to last forever? The fact that, heretofore, its causes and modes of prevention or of cure have been difficult to be understood by us, is no proof that they always will be so. Such a view seems to me only the time-honored objection of ultra conservatism, in its opposition, not only to progress itself, but even to the bare mention of it.

Since this report was first presented to the Massachusetts Medical Society, the very valuable volume, containing the Army Returns,* has given us details which sustain the position I have arrived at, although, by themselves, the law of development of phthisis I am contending for, could not have been ascertained.

In support of these assertions, I quote the following extracts from Dr. Coolidge's remarks, page 497.

"*First.* Temperature, considered by itself, does not exert that marked controlling influence on the development or progress of phthisis, which has been attributed to it. If a high range of temperature were favorable to the consumptive, the South Atlantic Region, the South Interior, East and Gulf Coast of Florida, should exhibit a lower ratio than the colder regions of the North and Northwest, whereas the contrary obtains; and again, if a high range of temperature were the controlling element in causing an increased ratio of this disease in the low southern regions above-named, we ought *not* to find a lower proportion of cases in Texas, where the temperature is higher, nor in the South Interior West, where it is nearly the same as in the South Atlantic Region.

"*Second.* The most important atmospherical condition for a consumptive is *dryness.* An examination of the rain tables will serve in *part* to elucidate this position, and in *part* only, for the total annual precipitation in rain and snow may be equal in two or more places, and yet the average condition of the air as respects moisture—the dew-point—may widely differ. It is impossible to represent all these differences by statistical tables, but the fact has been forcibly impressed upon the compiler during the minute examinations necessary to the preparation of this report.

"*Third.* Next to dryness, in importance, is an equable temperature, a temperature uniform for long periods, and not disturbed by sudden or frequent changes. A uniformly *low* temperature is much to be preferred to a uniformly *high* temperature. The former exerts a tonic and stimulating effect upon the general system, while the latter produces general debility and nervous exhaustion. The worst possible climate for a consumptive is one of long-continued high temperature and high dew-point."

Dr. Coolidge likewise gives the annexed table, with the following remarks:—

"With the exception of West Point (young men), the lowest rate of consumption occurs in New Mexico, and the highest in the South Atlantic Region. The South Interior East and the Gulf coast of Florida give the next highest proportion. The ratios for these regions, and also those for California, are higher than for any of the regions in the northern division."

---

* Statistical Report, &c., *ut supra.*

	Regions.	Mean Strength.	No. treated.	Deaths.	Ratio of cases to 1000 of Mean Str'gth.
1	Coast of New England	3,963	19	5	4.8
2	New York Harbor	9,387	56	35	5.9
3	West Point	6,901	6	8	.8
4	North Interior East	3,553	17	10	4.7
5	The Great Lakes	10,346	47	33	4.5
6	North Interior West	7,230	30	15	4.1
7	Middle Atlantic	6,299	16	14	2.5
8	Middle Interior East	2,456	6	3	2.4
9	Newport Barracks, Ky	1,454	5	4	3.4
10	Jefferson and St. Louis	5,580	23	21	4.1
11	Middle Interior West	5,319	28	13	5.2
12	South Atlantic	2,800	26	5	9.2
13	South Interior East	5,919	43	28	7.2
14	South Interior West	10,013	20	25	2.
15	Atlantic Coast, Florida	835	2	1	2.3
16	Gulf Coast, "	2,299	16	3	6.9
17	Texas, South Frontier	4,450	18	11	4.
18	Texas, Western "	6,324	25	12	3.9
19	New Mexico	5,873	8	3	1.3
20	California, Southern	1,707	9	5	5.2
21	California, Northern	1,599	9	4	5.6
22	Oregon, Washington	1,831	6	2	3.2

Dr. Coolidge remarks that the land east and from the base of the Rocky Mountains, and west of the Great Lakes, is favorable for consumptives.

Again, examination of the several regions shows, in a "marked degree, the effect of long-continued high temperature combined with excessive moisture (high dew-point) in the production and development of consumption." (Page 338.)

Since delivering the Address, I have received the following letters from two respected members of the Society. It will be seen that they hold exactly opposite views of the question in debate—one opposing it by special facts and general statements, the other sustaining it by statistics.

GROVELAND, May 30, 1862.

Dear Sir,—I am not certain whether I have made any response to your Circulars on the subject of consumption, as I should have done; but presuming that you are glad of facts at any time, I sit down to give you a series of such as have come under my observation, during a practice of forty-eight years.

My circle of practice is over as great a diversity of soil and elevation as can probably be found, within the same extent of land, in the State. High hills, sandy plains, a tide-water river, quick streams, a clear pond of three hundred acres, and a boggy pond and wide meadows. It would give me great pleasure to conduct you over the town, and have you locate the spots for consumption. It does appear to me that you would find it difficult to apply your theory to the facts, as they have arisen under my observation.

I have never supposed the vicinity of a clear running stream unhealthy, and I have seen nothing to shake that belief. I live twenty-five rods from the Merrimack, and thirty feet above it. I have brought up eight children;

none consumptive. ——— was an invalid when married, forty-eight years ago, and has lived here forty-five years. She has *adhesions* from pleurisy, but is about her cares now, aged seventy-two! We have now 1,400 inhabitants in town, perhaps 1,100 on an average all the time (forty-four years), with about twenty deaths a year, and, as near as I can calculate, not much over one a year by consumption. On a street directly on the river bank, of about 200 inhabitants, we have now, I believe, 17 past 70 years of age, and one over 90.

On a mill-stream, which passes a mile from the great pond to the river, in eleven of the newest houses, there has been one case of consumption.

On a dry knoll, half a mile from the river, and forty feet above a clear running stream, a young man, aged 22, with long-lived ancestry, lately died of consumption.

Along the river bank, thirty years ago, three young people, a brother and two sisters, died of consumption; the parents now living—near 80, and other children healthy.

On a high, dry spot, a mile from the river, a lady, aged 75, lately died of consumption; near by, her husband's parents lived to about 90. Her husband lived to be 75, but died of *rum.*

On a low spot, by the side of a brook and meadow, D. H. lived to 91; daughter on the spot, now 70; brother died about 75.

On a high, dry, sandy soil, fifty rods from the mill-stream, and sixty feet above it, P. C., aged 60, and two sons, 16 to 20, died with consumption.

On a dry plain, near a mile from the river, E. R. died of consumption, aged about 60; wife living now, aged 92; children healthy. A few rods distant, on as dry a spot, H. N., a girl of 12, died of consumption.

On a low spot, near the level of a meadow, but the house on a dry spot, B. H. and wife now live, near 80.

On a dry spot, but near a swamp and often stagnant water, Rev. W. B. lived to be 92; his son to about 80; his grandson, now living, 96; his mother was over 90; the families that grew up, and went out from the spot, healthy and long lived.

A house near this, and nearer to the meadow, has had but one death by consumption in the two families which have resided there, in forty-five years. A girl born there died, ten or twelve years old, with consumption, consequent upon whooping cough and measles; the mother died with consumption, after removing for twenty years to a much higher and drier spot.

On a dry spot, but near a meadow and mill-stream, M. P., Esq., and wife, near sixty years ago, buried three children, 12 to 20 years old, with consumption. He lived to be 80, and the wife to be 90, and no more consumption in the family through two generations born and brought up there.

In a high and dry neighborhood, well known for its health, and beautiful location, S. S., a fine girl of 20, died of consumption twenty-five years ago; her mother, aged 75, died of consumption. Lately a nephew to the first named, brought up there, and residing there except when at Amherst College and Andover Institution, died of consumption; all of which places, of birth and residence, might have been selected for their beautiful and healthy location. A sister of the first named, married 30 years ago, and living in the worst locality in this town, on account of its contiguous meadow, a tan-yard, and being liable to the filtration of a cemetery 30 rods off, on much higher ground, is living, aged 60, though probably tuberculous.

Dr. P., half a mile from the river, and 100 feet above it, lost his second son at 18, by consumption. His eldest son, the late Dr. W. T. P———, of S—— B——, died at Jamaica Plain, of consumption. The Doctor, sen., died in 1845, aged 87; his wife, about 1850, aged 65, with consumption.

Some have accused the river of producing fevers, but I do not find ground for the charge. I think as many die in Georgetown, my native place, directly back of this town, as here.

I have no doubt that stagnant water, with decaying vegetables, is unhealthy; but running streams, or ponds with clean shores, I think not.

On our river road, two and a half miles, with nearly 600 people, I can make out but 20 cases of tubercular consumption. I omit cases of decay at 70, 80 and 90 years, unless with distinct lung disease; also cases of dropsy and intemperance. Within the same limits I can name 47 persons now living, or who died, over 80, and 4 over 90.

We have very few fogs on the Merrimack. I have resided on the Connecticut River, and should think there are ten foggy mornings there to one here. We have five or six feet flow of tide, but it is by the backing up of the river current. We never have salt water within four or five miles of this place.

Consumption is often hereditary, and marches on with steady tread to take its victims; nor does locality seem to have much to do with it. Your late patient, H—— N——, of G———, was an instance. His grandfather and grandmother died of consumption; his mother, an uncle, and, I think, three aunts, died of consumption; his own sister, and a half sister by the mother, ditto, under my care. Two own cousins, viz., the late C—— A——, Esq., of B———, and a brother in Minnesota, both lately died of consumption, aged 26 and 28. These were all my relations and friends.

With the highest respect for your medical and scientific ability, I must think that my experience would not fully sustain your views.

JEREMIAH SPOFFORD.

I thank Dr. Spofford for his early and earnest reply to the Address. The statement of his long experience is valuable. Yet it does not, of course, induce me to reject the results I have drawn from a wide correspondence with his and my colleagues, in all quarters of the State. I have never claimed that locality is the *sole* cause of consumption. The hereditary nature of the complaint, in many cases, cannot be denied. I have explicitly stated, in the Address, that I do not *know* of any spot in New England in which consumption has been proved not to exist. All these admissions, and they are all that the letter requires, are consistent with the belief that a house situated on a damp soil is, in any part of New England, generally from that fact, much more liable to have consumption prevail in it, than if it were situated on a drier place; and that in some way, to us unknown, the location and consumption stand in the relation of cause and effect. It would gratify me very much, if Dr. Spofford would give the exact amount of deaths by consumption, and by all diseases, and the population, in various distinctly different regions of his town, as marked by different degrees of moisture of the soil, so that they might be exactly compared in reference to this question. Perhaps he would be led, by such data, to different conclusions from those advanced in his letter, and become convinced, as Dr. Hovey of Atkinson and others have been, in spite of their previous and decided *general impressions.**

---

* See Address, pages 13, 51.

The second letter, as follows, from Dr. Appleton, sustains the views of the Address—giving, in fact, nearly three times as many cases, in proportion to the population, in the wet districts as the dry. It will be remembered that Dr. Appleton gave, formerly, statistics from West Newbury.* Those given in his present letter fully sustain his previous statements.

Boston, June 6, 1862.

My Dear Sir,—In the prosecution of your researches into the prevalence of consumption in Massachusetts, as affected by the humidity or dryness of different localities, you may be interested in the results afforded by the registry of deaths in West Newbury, for the last seven years, which corroborate and strengthen the conclusions, derived from the statistics of the ten preceding years, which are already in your possession.

The population of the town has not varied greatly since the last census, but has rather diminished within the last year, in consequence of the general depression of business occasioned by the war.

The whole number of deaths in the town for the seven years, from 1855 to 1861, inclusive, is 242; of which 59 are registered as from consumption. A reference to the map of the town, which was prepared to illustrate the statistics of deaths from 1845 to 1855, and in which the boundaries of the school districts are described, will show the great proportion of cases in the three northern, or what may be classed as the moist districts.

The deaths from consumption in West Newbury, from 1855 to 1861, were as follows:

In District No. 1,	8	In District No. 4,	3
2,	17	5,	3
3,	27	6,	1
			59

In the three northern (moister, river) districts, 52 in 1271 population, or 1 in every 24.42 persons.

In the three southern (drier, warmer) districts, 7 in 475, or 1 in every 67.85 persons.

It is possible that some of the deaths, which are registered as from consumption, may have taken place from other causes; but I think that this will not affect the general result in regard to the proportion of deaths in each district.

I will now call your attention to a single locality in the western part of district No. 2, a plan of which I have attempted to represent in the accompanying sketch. "Main Street," in West Newbury, is built upon an elevated ridge, nearly parallel with the Merrimack River, at a distance generally of more than half a mile from the stream, and, at this point, elevated at least 150 feet above the level. The soil is a clayey loam, with a subsoil of clay, retaining the moisture, the cellars of the houses which have been excavated here, generally containing water in the winter and spring. With the exception of the house marked A on the plan, which was built about sixty years since, all the tenements represented north of this street have been erected within ten years, "Prospect Street" having been laid out in 1853. The ground, over which this street is located, falls rapidly towards the north, and towards a tract of moist land which must retain much of the surface drainage of the more elevated portion. (See plan.)

---

* See Table IV. in Address; also note to the same.

In five of the houses, represented on the plan, and designated as B, C, D, E and F, seven of the seventeen deaths, which occurred in the district from consumption, took place between 1855 and 1861. Two persons died in each of the houses B and C, and one each in D, E and F. There are also at the present time, in D, two members of the family who exhibit unequivocal symptoms of phthisis.

I have not the requisite data at hand to enable me to give the percentage of deaths to the population of the several districts.

Hoping that the facts I have communicated will be of sufficient interest to justify the prolixity of the letter,

I remain, very truly yours,

J. APPLETON.

Dr. Bowditch.

ERRATA.

In Table IV., the statistics for Townsend should have been more definitely arranged, as follows :

In Dry Localities.	In Localities of medium Moisture.	In clayey Subsoil, retaining Moisture.	In Low and Damp Places.
16.36	19.11	25.85	30.85

On page 21, second paragraph, "in *three* instances" should have been in *a few* instances.

In third paragraph, "twenty-one" should be twenty.

In fourth paragraph, "a little *more* than one third" should be a little *less*, &c.

In quoting Dr. Cotting's tables, and in my remarks thereupon (pp. 66–67 Address — 94 Appendix), I did not deem it necessary to verify the tables ; but a friend draws my attention to a serious arithmetical error in the adding of the first column in Dr. Cotting's "Table of the Locality of Deaths by Consumption." In that table, the total of deaths by consumption in the "high" places for four years is given as 170 ; whereas it should have been 130. Therefore, in his prefatory remarks upon this table, Dr. Cotting, instead of claiming that "those who died of consumption on high and dry lands, amount to 170, or two thirds of the whole number," should have stated 130, or a little more than one half of the whole number (257). This, it will be perceived, makes a vast difference, and evidently tends not in the least to disprove, but rather to sustain, the doctrines of the Address, and my own special remarks on this part of Dr. Cotting's paper. For certainly, Dr. Cotting cannot claim that any near approximation to *one half*, or even one third of the population of Roxbury reside on "the low, wet or made lands."

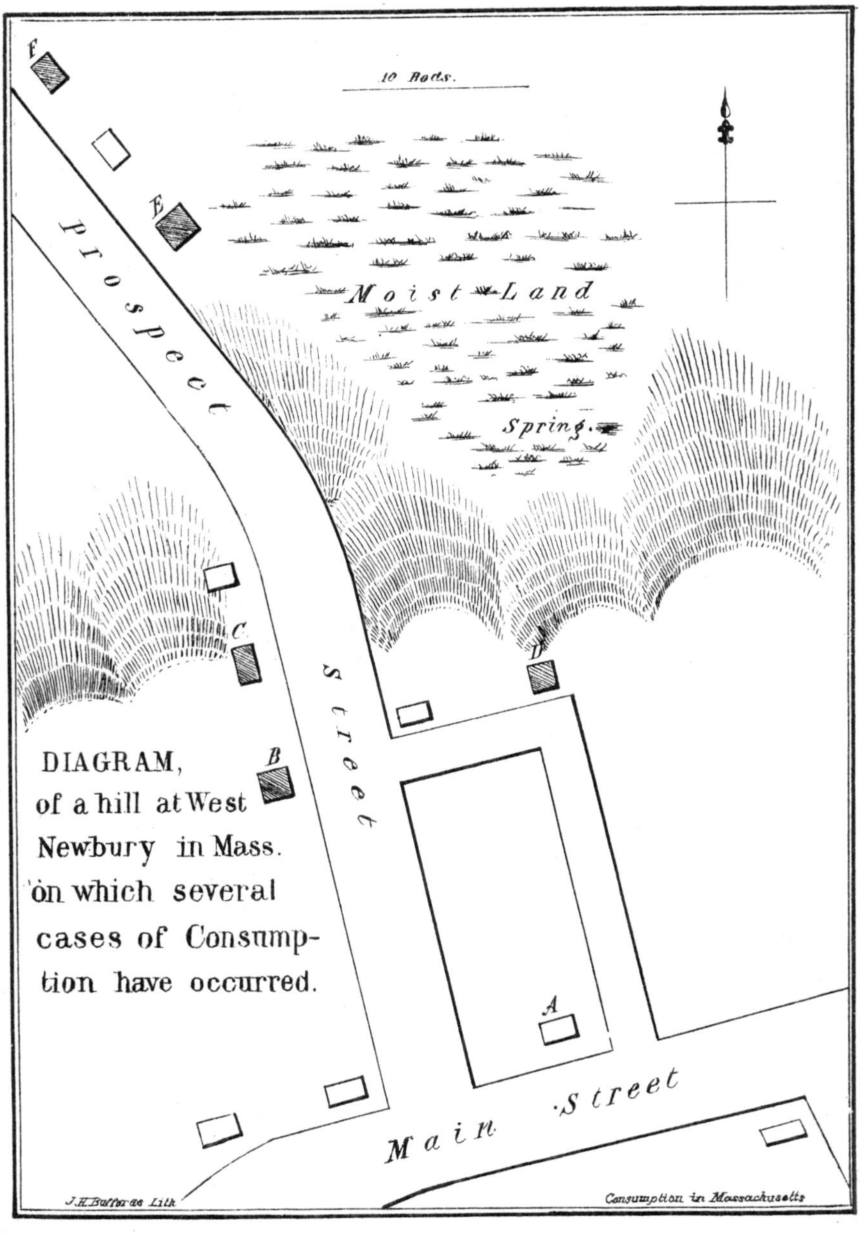

DIAGRAM,
of a hill at West Newbury in Mass. on which several cases of Consumption have occurred.

IS CONSUMPTION EVER CONTAGIOUS,

OR

COMMUNICATED BY ONE PERSON TO ANOTHER IN ANY MANNER?

A PAPER PREPARED FOR THE BOSTON SOCIETY FOR MEDICAL OBSERVATION.

BY

HENRY I. BOWDITCH, M.D.

PROFESSOR OF CLINICAL MEDICINE IN HARVARD UNIVERSITY.

BOSTON:

PRINTED BY DAVID CLAPP.....334 WASHINGTON STREET.

1864.

IS CONSUMPTION EVER CONTAGIOUS,

OR COMMUNICATED BY ONE PERSON TO ANOTHER IN ANY MANNER?

THIS question may seem one of very little importance, because we all may be of one opinion, viz., in favor of the negative of the proposition. Yet it is one about which I have been interested, in consequence of some cases that have fallen under my notice during the last ten or fifteen years. These cases I shall relate to the Society; but before doing so, let me refer briefly to the views of the medical profession on this topic, historically considered. In all that relates to medical opinion previous to the present century, I shall depend on the learned work by Dr. Young.* It would seem, from Dr. Young's statements, that all the chief authors who, previously to the last quarter of the last century, treated of the subject, were full believers in the contagiousness of consumption. It is also well known, that public opinion, which is always the reflection of a preceding medical opinion, sustained that view, at least in the southern portions of Europe. The Italians, until a very recent date, have had certain quarantine and other regulations relative to those dying of this disease, as are common now in smallpox cases. Aristotle, according to Dr. Mason Good, states that this belief in the contagiousness of the disease was common among the Greeks. Galen regarded it as unwise to pass even a day with a consumptive. Morton†, 1619, Riverius,‡ 1656, and above all, a century later, the learned and sagacious Morgagni,§ 1761, would not dissect a phthisical patient's

---

* Practical and Historical Treatise on Consumptive Diseases, deduced from Original Observations and collected from Authors of all Ages. By Thomas Young, M.D., F.R.S., London, 1815.

† Morton. Phthisiologia, London, 1619, p. 185.

‡ Riverius. Opera Medica, Fol. Geneva, 1728, d. 1656, &c.

§ De Causis et Sedibus Morborum, Fol. Venice, 1761, Ex. xix., 53—xlix., 15.

body because of the risk he thought would be run of taking the disease. Dr. Withering,* in 1775, claims that it is certainly infectious.

Subsequently to this long period of almost entire faith in the contagiousness of the disease, we have a period of doubt and of questioning upon the subject for about twenty-five or thirty years.

Dr. Cullen,† in 1777, dares not assert that it is never contagious, especially in warm climates, but he had never seen a case, in which it was decidedly communicated by one individual to another.

The Edinburgh professor evidently doubted the commonly received opinion, but was unwilling to take a bold stand against the idea of contagiousness, as those of the same school did in 1794 (i. e.. seventeen years afterwards), who not only opposed the notion, but presented strong cases against it.‡

Dr. T. Reid,§ of London, 1782, allows that, in extreme cases, it may be slightly contagious, and young persons should not sleep in the same room with a phthisical patient.

During the same year, 1782, Bursieri‖ says the Colleges of Physicians of Tuscany had declared their disbelief in its contagiousness; but this did not prevent government from taking precautions against it.

Emale,¶ 1783, thinks it so contagious that it is dangerous to draw milk from the breasts of a woman, as recommended by Chevillard and others, for the cure of consumption, for fear of the disease being given to the nurse.

Vogel,** 1785, is quite convinced of its contagiousness.

Darwin,†† 1793, is a complete believer of its contagiousness, in *persons nearly allied.*

By these quotations—coupled with the fact that I find none, during the same period, decidedly opposed to the proposition—I think I have given some proof—first, of the very general consent to the proposition of the contagious nature of consumption, until the commencement of the last quarter of the last century; second, that from that time until about 1800, there was evidently great indecision. From 1800, with some very few exceptions, Medical Opinion and Public Opinion have been gradually becoming settled in opposition to the theory of contagion. No one will deny that Morgagni showed great weakness in being unwilling to dissect the body of a phthisical patient. In fact, no one would hesitate to regard the disease, as seen now, wholly innocuous to the degree feared by the great pathologist of the last century.

* Account of the Foxglove. Birmingham, 1785.
† First Lines of the Practice of Physic, Edinb. 1777.
‡ Dr. Young. Supra, p. 360.
§ Essay on Nature and Cure of Phthisis Pulmonalis. Lond. 1782.
‖ J. B. Bursieri. Institutiones Medicinæ Practicæ, 4 v. Venice, 1782. English by Brown. 4 v. Edinb. 1800.
¶ Emale. Journal Médicale, lxiii. 1783.
** S. C. Vogel. Handbuch der Practischen Arzney-Wissenshaft. 1785.
†† T. Beddoes to E. Darwin, on a New Method of treating Consumption.

I may here remark that one wonders at the fears of Morgagni, when he remembers that Fabricius Hildanus describes several examinations of bodies of persons dying of consumption, and this more than a century before Morgagni lived.

The following resumé of the authorities on the subject since 1793 up to the present time, will include my third period, or that of nearly utter denial of the idea of contagion in connection with consumption.

Only two writers of note and of undoubtedly strong minds, and these Americans, can be found to defend the proposition of contagiousness. These two writers are nearly at the two extremities of the period now under consideration, viz.: Benjamin Rush,* 1793, and Drake,† 1854—about a half a century later. Dr. Rush is fully convinced of the contagiousness of the disease, and quotes what I cannot but think rather apocryphal cases sustaining his views. Dr. Drake, without taking the affirmative decidedly, nevertheless evidently leans very strongly towards it; quotes facts, and argues analogically that such a proposition is quite in accordance with the fitness of things.

Meanwhile a certain number, especially in the earlier part of the century, are in doubt. Dr. Heberden,‡ for example, 1802, has not been able to make up a decided opinion upon the subject; but he had seen several cases in which he could not find any more plausible reason than contagion, from the patient having been constantly in attendance on another, and even sleeping in the same room. The very same year, Haygarth§ and Darwin‖ decided against the proposition.

Wilson,¶ 1803, says it is rarely attributable to contagion, but it is wisest to avoid sleeping with a consumptive patient. Little is said by authors upon the subject till 1809; and from that period up to the present time, authorities may, with the exception of the two first (viz., Rush and Drake), be classed either as being in doubt, and, at times, very decided opposition to the idea of contagion; or they ignore the whole subject, and thus virtually seem to consider it beneath their notice.

In the first class we find Portal,** 1809; Laennec,†† 1818; Cowan,‡‡ 1835; Davies,§§ 1835; Ancel,‖‖ 1852; Watson¶¶, 1857; and

---

* Medical Inquiries, 1793.

† Diseases of the Interior Valley of North America. 1854, Vol. 2.

‡ Commentarii de Morborum historia et curatione. Lond. 1802.

§ Haygarth. Young, p. 395.

‖ T. Beddoes. Hygeia, or Essays Moral and Physical. Bristol, 1802.

¶ A. P. Wilson. Treatise on Febrile Diseases, 1803.

** Portal. Observations sur la Nature et le Traitement de la Pleuro-Pneumonie. Paris, 1808.

†† Laennec. L'Auscultation Médiate. Paris, 1818.

‡‡ Cowan. Translation of Louis on Phthisis. London, 1835.

§§ T. Davies. Lectures on Diseases of the Lungs and Heart. Lond. 1835.

‖‖ H. Ancel. Treatise on Tuberculosis, the Constitutional Origin of Consumption and Scrofula. Lond. 1852.

¶¶ Thomas Watson. Lectures on the Principles and Practice of Physic. London, 1857.

Cotton,* 1858. All these writers actually oppose the notion. Dr. Watson rather dogmatically would settle the question by declaring that "a *diathesis* cannot be contagious."

In the second class are found the following well-known authors, most of whom have written special treatises on tuberculosis, and some of them have gone quite elaborately into the causes of consumption. Louis,† 1825; C. J. B. Williams,‡ 1834; Stokes,§ 1843; Blakiston,‖ 1848; Copland;¶ Bennett,** 1858; Lawson,†† 1861; Todd,‡‡ 1861.

From these quotations it is evident that, at the present time, we may say that Medical and Public Opinion are almost the exact reverse of what they were previously to the middle of the last century. My own doubts have disappeared under the close examination of my own cases, and of those reported by others. Nevertheless, I should not agree with the extremes of either party, but should hold, that while there is no positive proof of the real contagiousness of consumption, it would be very unwise to deny that some cases do arise, in which a close attendance upon and devotion to persons affected with phthisis is the prominent exciting cause of tuberculous disease of the lungs, in persons apparently healthy.

Similar views are held by others. In proof, I quote as follows: John Hogg,§§ 1860, remarks it is difficult to say if contagion can be fairly classed among the causes of consumption; but, he adds, it would be the *acmé* of imprudence to place a young person, not perhaps in the best of health herself, in close attendance on or near another. To this last expression of opinion I should give my adhesion, but I would not limit the remark to those who are not in good health—for I think our cases bear out the assertion that it is hazardous for even the most healthy to run that risk. A similar opinion is also held by Mons. Gueneau de Mussy,‖‖ clinical successor to Chomel, in Paris. He declares, 1864, wholly against contagion, as usually understood, but at the same time believes that it is probably transmitted by coition and by very intimate relations with an individual during any of the periods of the disease. At the time of writing he had two cases in the wards of Hotel Dieu. He quotes Andral as coinciding with him. He has observed a trouble in the throat among

* R. Payne Cotton. On Consumption, its Nature, &c. London, 1858.
† P. C. H. Louis. Sur la Phthisie. Paris, 1825.
‡ C. J. B. Williams. Physical Signs of Diseases of the Chest. Am. Ed., 1834.
§ W. Stokes. Diseases of the Chest. 2d Am. Ed., 1844.
‖ G. Peyton Blakiston. Practical Observations on Diseases of the Chest. London. Am. Edition, 1848.
¶ Medical Dictionary. Article, Tubercular Consumption.
** J. H. Bennett. Clinical Lectures. American Edition. New York, 1858.
†† L. M. Lawson. Practical Treatise on Pulmonary Consumption. Cincinnati, 1861.
‡‡ R. B. Todd. Clinical Lectures. London, 1861.
§§ John Hogg. Practical Observations on the Prevention of Consumption. London, 1860.
‖‖ Leçons sur les causes et le traitement de la tuberculose pulmonaire. Hotel Dieu, Union Medicale, vol. 4, p. 374, Nov., 1859.

those who live with the tuberculous. He thinks it more common for consumption to be transmitted from a man to a woman than from a woman to a man.

These general statements give a glance, at least, at the three periods of opinion, and the commencement of a fourth, on this subject; viz., 1st, the period of almost undoubting faith—extending from the earliest records of medicine up to 1775, or thereabout; 2d, a short period, of 25 or 30 years, of great and painful doubt; 3d, a time of utter scepticism; and, 4th, perhaps I may add, a modified faith, not coinciding with either the "everlasting Yea," "the centre of indifference," or "everlasting Nay," as Carlyle would express it.

Let me proceed now to the examination of my own cases.

Case I.—A gentleman died Feb. 13, 1858, after two years' illness, with confirmed and undoubted phthisis. I saw him and examined him, and know that he had all the marked rational and physical phenomena of the disease.

The wife consulted me March 4, 1864, with decided signs of phthisis. It appears that her family was usually quite healthy. Parents alive: mother 56 years old, asthmatic; father well. One uncle, by the father's side, had died of consumption. She was an only child, and had always been, up to the time of her husband's illness, in most robust health. In fact, she never "dreamed of being ill," either generally or locally. She was her husband's sole nurse during his year's illness. She slept with him to the last. He complained if she left him. He wanted the warmth of her body to keep off his chills at night. Often her clothing was wet by the moisture from his body. Her parents protested against this course, and warned her of the consequences; but the wish expressed by the husband, her own confidence in her own health, and abandonment of all thought of self for her husband's sake; these considerations overcame all others, and she continued this course until the end of his life. When this time arrived, she found herself wholly worn down, and she had never been well afterwards. She had been much less capable of endurance, and was easily fatigued by comparatively light work. Every spring she had been worse than at other portions of the year. She had had severe cough from the first, with aggravations of it at times, but with only slight sputa. A year since, hæmoptysis occurred—about ʒ i., bright, arterial. She had had more or less pain about the right shoulder; had been able to lie on either side, and had never been seriously prostrated. Her hæmoptysis occurred after the performance of a very difficult piece of music, requiring extra physical exertion and mental attention. She had had at times some dyspnœa; no palpitation, but was easily tired by walking. Her appetite had been fair, with good digestion as its attendant. Menses regular—urine variable, at times very light colored. She had had a series of periods of emaciation, and subsequently some gaining of flesh, but with a gradual loss of 25 pounds—having fallen from 150 to 125, her present weight. Chills and heat, but no sweating had occurred. This spring, for the first time, she had had hoarseness, and coughed, morning and evening, in paroxysms of about half an hour. She had taken iron and other tonics with benefit, and whiskey not regularly. When I saw her, her countenance was a little pale, not much emaciated, or showing the marks of severe disease. Pulse 88. Tongue clean. The physical signs were as follows:—There was flatness behind right clavicle, and dry crackling to the fourth rib. Voice a little resonant. Flatness also at the top of the right back, and a coarse crackle and slight resonance of voice. Rales, though less marked, even to the base of the lung, and respiratory murmur rather rough even there. Respiration in left lung noisy, somewhat sibilous.

She evidently had tubercles, slowly developing, at the top of the right lung. She considered that this was the culmination of a disease excited by her close attention to her husband during his illness. The facts of the mother's "asthma," and the uncle's death by phthisis, may throw some doubt as to the contact with her husband being the chief cause of the disease in her case. She was hereditarily (so the sceptics will say) tending to phthisical disease—and the over-exertion, &c., broke her down, and made her an easy victim.

I might, in reply, say, that if we take the simple fact of one uncle having died of phthisis as a proof of the *hereditary* disposition, and this in opposition to a most perfectly robust health up to the time of beginning to attend her husband, I cannot but think as much may be said of almost every family. There is scarcely one in this community in which some member, remote it may be, has not had symptoms of phthisis. The "*asthma*" of the mother does not really bear upon the subject of *her phthisis*.

Case II.—Miss E., a young and very healthy-looking woman, I saw in November, 1855. She was the sole attendant of a very sick, tuberculous husband, and slept with him during all the periods of his disease. I was struck with her apparently robust health. A short time after her husband's death she had hæmoptysis. She is now, I believe, alive and married again, but is ill with phthisis, which commenced then, but which makes, however, very slow progress, and does not seem to very *materially* impair her health.

Case III.—In 1855 I attended Mr. H., who was an invalid with pleurisy, and subsequently tubercular disease appeared. He remained for years, fighting against the complaint, and finally died with tubercular pneumothorax. His wife's mother died of phthisis, but she herself was splendid in her kind of robust English form, when her husband fell ill. She *devoted* herself without stint to him, and gradually began to "heck." On examination, physical signs were noticed under the clavicle. The symptoms rapidly increased, and she died before her husband, and was evidently tuberculous.

Those knowing the facts believe, as I believe, that if she had not attended upon him so closely and so long, she might be now alive.

CASE IV.—Miss S. sprung from a family, in which no trace of consumption is known ever to have existed. She was living as a farmer's daughter on a most healthy site, and enjoyed most strong and robust health, when she went to attend an invalid friend, to whom she was most tenderly attached. The friendship was mutual. The invalid sought for and received the closest attention on the part of her young companion. They slept in adjacent rooms at night, and the strong one acted as nurse at all hours, day and night. This attendance commenced in July, 1853, and continued till June, 1854, eleven months, when, at the request of her parents, our patient went home. In August, however, she again spent a week with her friend, and was with her at her death, August 30, 1854. During all this period the invalid did not wish any one else to do aught for her, and her young companion often lifted her when the patient was too feeble to raise herself. During one of these efforts Miss S. felt that she had "strained herself." Ever after she had an uncomfortable "coldness" at the epigastrium and a tendency to chilliness—with, subsequently, in the spring of 1855, some dyspepsia. In the following months, her parents noticed her rather feeble condition, but did not regard her as seriously ill. She was treated as a dyspeptic, and considered herself as such. She had scarlet fever in the spring. In August, 1855, cough set in, i. e. after twelve months' invalidism, and the cough continued uninterruptedly till death. Diarrhœa commenced in March, 1856. She died of phthisis, July 27th, 1856, nearly two years after her friend's decease. I saw her once in the spring of 1856. She then had the signs of anomalous tuberculosis, i. e. crepitus, a pure tubular respiration, and solidification of the lower two thirds of the right lung. She also had had two abscesses under the arms, a few days before my visit.

CASE V.—A gentleman whom I was attending in advanced phthisis, in 1855, assured me that, though one brother had died of phthisis, after some particular exposure, he did not deem himself hereditarily disposed to the disease, as no other case had occurred in the family. This gentleman attended constantly on his wife, who died of phthisis. On my asking whether he thought that attendance had had any influence on his own health, he remarked instantly, as if the idea had previously occurred to him, that the *first* marked paroxysm of coughing he had ever had, and from which he dated all his own ills, was when he was raising his wife in bed and inhaled very deeply her breath. It caused much irritation at the time, and coughing was produced, which continued afterwards.

CASE VI.—Mrs. ——— I saw, October, 1854, aged 30 years. She had been taken suddenly with hæmoptysis. She had had five attacks of the same previously—the first at 18 years of age. Usually they had been of slight duration, and in the interval her health had been excellent. She had slight disease at the top of both lungs. She had been the sole attendant of her husband, who had died about two years previously of phthisis. She had often risen in the night and given him her warm and dry night dress, and moved him to her side of the bed, while she lay down upon the mattress, wet with his sweat, and with only a blanket thrown over it. This was only one of the numerous acts of self-sacrifice which she performed. She told me she knew she was running a risk, but she did not, at that time, care for it. From the time of her husband's death her own health had been materially changed—she had never been as well as before. After contending against the disease ten years, and being at times able to labor much, as superintendent of a large mantilla establishment, she is now in a hopeless state of disease. But she is fully convinced that the close attention to her husband first undermined her health.

CASE VII.—Mrs. ———. This is doubtful as to present diagnosis—but I fear phthisis will result. She has no hereditary tendency, and is a stout, full built woman, and was, till lately, healthy. She attended her husband, who died of phthisis in June last, 1863, after nine months' illness. She was his sole nurse. She slept with him till the last, and scarcely left his room for three or four months preceding his death. She was, of course, fatigued, but went into the country and felt sufficiently well, except she had a liability to headache, to which she was not subject before. In November or December, 1863, she first noticed some dyspnœa; afterwards some palpitation and some sweating at night. These symptoms increased, and she was thought to have phthisis. I found evidence of latent pleuritic effusion filling the whole of the left chest. Tapping was performed Feb. 9, 1864, with relief to the dyspnœa. Between three and four pints of serous fluid was drawn out, but there has been no frank improvement of the local signs. The lung has never freely expanded, but, on the contrary, dulness has always remained, and only the finest crepitus or cough is produced at upper part of lung.

May 14, 1864.—Since this was written, the lung has expanded more, and the fluid that remained has been absorbed. There is, however, still an obscurity of murmur and much less resonance than usual.

CASE VIII.—I saw two sisters in the central part of Massachusetts. I visited them in October, 1863. The parents cough. The grandmother, by the mother's side, had two aunts and a sister die of consumption. Evidently the disease strongly tends to occur in the family. One of the present sisters was dying of advanced tuberculous disease; she had had slight cough for two years, but only broke down two months before I saw her, and apparently from overexposure, at a celebration on the return of soldiers to her native town, she being chief manager. The whole of left lung had the fine crepitus of recent tubercles, and there were signs of a few at the top of the right. The sister was devoted to her, and declared she would not leave her. She watched with her, and would not take even the slightest precaution. I warned her of danger, but she paid no heed, careless of everything save attention to the sick one.

The physician has written to me, within the past six weeks, that she, too, is beginning to show signs of phthisis, and is, in reality, more rapidly sinking than her sister.

CONCLUSIONS, FROM THESE CASES.

Out of the 8, we have 7 females, viz., 5 wives, 1 sister, 1 female friend; and only 1 male.

They may be divided into three classes, according to their hereditary tendency to phthisis.

1st.	Possibly, phthisical tendencies previous to exposure, though apparently healthy at commencement of attendance,	5
2d.	No such tendencies,	2
3d.	Doubtful, but appeared healthy,	1

In 1st class, only one had had symptoms previously, viz., hæmoptysis, years previously, without serious influence on the health. In the four others, one or more members of the family had had phthisis; viz., one mother, one uncle, one brother, and one sister.

The opponents of the idea that contagion had anything to do with the production of phthisis in the 1st and also in the 3d class, viz., in six of the eight cases given, will argue that these cases are utterly worthless as a ground-work of any argument for contagion, and therefore they should be put wholly out of the question. I cannot entirely agree to this view of the subject, when I remember that, without exception, my patients were all, apparently, in good health before they fell under the supposed deleterious influence of close attendance upon the consumptive friend; and that from the termination of that attendance the health of all was found to be undermined. Hence I really think I can claim, with a certain degree of reason, that, whatever were the hereditary tendencies, the attentions in nursing the phthisical friends were the *exciting* cause of their own disease.

But let us examine the two remaining cases:—And here also we must admit a certain lameness in one of them as a basis of argument, viz., a doubt about the *certainty* of the diagnosis. So we are really reduced to only one perfectly reliable case, in which no trace of tuberculosis can be found previously to the exposure. Now in this case, if we can ever allow ourselves to speak of causes in diseases, the phthisis and subsequent death were not only a sequence, but I think and others think a veritable consequence, in the strictest relation of cause and effect, of her previous close attendance on a tuberculous patient. But was there necessarily contagion in this case? By no means, the anti-contagionists will reply. It may well be questioned whether anything at all similar to contagion, as we usually understand that term, can be predicated of it. There is proof enough of weakened health, of dyspepsia, and its usual concomitants, and after months of gradually deteriorating health phthisis did set in. But then the same result might have occurred without any attendance on any body. It is the most common way for phthisis to develope itself. Confinement in any bad atmosphere, ill ventilated apartments, anxiety and depression of mind, irregular digestion, have often produced identically the same results. Then, again, they may say—If contagion had anything really to do with it, why did it prove so long in showing itself? Usually contagion shows itself soon. This was months in developing itself.

Dr. Drake meets this argument, by saying that we really know nothing of the length of time necessary for the incubation of phthisical influences. One disease is promptly contagious, and runs its course rapidly. This is no reason that the same rapid course should be pursued in phthisis. On the contrary, all *its* phases are slow. Why not its period of incubation? In fact, have we not a proof of this in the years that pass over before an hereditary tendency bursts forth? The arguments against contagion drawn from the long period elapsing between exposure and the evident disease is therefore really of small moment. But it falls wholly, when we remember how hydrophobia and other deleterious influences may remain dormant for an indefinite length of time—how miasmatic influences may remain years unknown, and then suddenly show themselves.

But again, say the anti-contagionists, the nature of consumption is very different, certainly, from the majority of contagious diseases; there is no eruption as in smallpox, measles, scabies, syphilis, &c. Above all, the actual inoculations by Kostum, Le Pelletier, &c., proved abortive.

To this the contagionists might reply—But there is whooping-cough, mumps, some sore throats, pleuro-pneumonia in animals, &c., from which there is not apparently any morbific matter recognizable by the senses. Yet these are capable of producing their kind. In regard to actual experiments of inoculation, it is asserted that they were not satisfactorily performed.

Still further, the non-contagionists say—If contagion acts, why have we not had more cases in these many years, and why such a vast preponderance of married females amongst these patients? Does contagion usually select women? Why not rather suppose that the entire *abandon* with which women throw themselves into the duty of nursing; their total recklessness, at times, when attending on a dear friend, of the commonest rules of hygiene in regard to air, exercise, food and sleep—that these, conjoined with and acting upon an excessively sensitive nervous nature, are the causes of the disease in those cases?

We may thus argue pro and con upon the subject, and yet not arrive at exact and definite opinions, as to the precise matter in dispute; and I will close this part of my paper with the single remark, that the strongest argument I know against contagion, is the fact that, considering my facts at least, woman is more liable than man to be taken. Why this, if there be not something at any rate more important than contagion to explain the phenomena of the case? The really contagious disease spares neither age nor sex. There must be something, therefore, more than mere contagion.

FINAL STATEMENT OF VIEWS.

Let me say that I commenced this investigation strongly prepossessed with the idea (gained while attending my patients and with a cursory knowledge of their antecedents) of the essentially contagious nature of phthisis, under certain circumstances. The force of my own facts, when thoroughly examined, has led me materially to doubt the correctness of my former impressions.

I will lay down the following propositions, which I believe correct.

First.—Consumption is not *contagious* in the usual acceptation of that word.

Second.—It may be *infectious*, and to this extent only. By long attendance of the closest kind, by inhaling the breath of the phthisical patient, by living in the phthisical atmosphere, so to speak, and in general by a neglect of hygienic laws during such attendance, the health may be undermined and phthisis set in. How far the depressing passions may have an effect, it may be impossible to say; but that they exert an important and deleterious influence, we cannot deny. Doubtless the want of exercise and the neglect of all hygienic laws have an immense influence. But as we see all these influences, except the supposed infection, existing often, for a long time, without producing phthisis (for example, a long attendance on patients ill with other non-tubercular diseases), I do believe that, in some few instances at least, we must admit a degree of real infection in our estimate of the matter. Especially must we take this into consideration in the case of a sister or a brother in a family, where the hereditary tendency to phthisis is strong; for in this case I doubt whether it would be safe to allow the sister to attend as nurse, even with the best moral and physical hygienic influences.

I am confirmed in this view by two more considerations. We see carcinoma and other chronic diseases have never even suggested this idea of contagion to the medical profession, at least so strongly as phthisis has. Is not this an argument in favor of the idea of there being something peculiar in tubercle, whereby it is capable, at certain periods of its development, of producing its kind? Second, I deem of some importance the positive statement made to me by a husband, the sole male patient among our cases. He distinctly asserted that the first real cough arose when he was raising his wife in bed, and consequently was making an effort and drew in a deep breath, inhaling at the moment while his wife was exhaling. The chief part of the air he drew in was loaded with emanations from her lungs. As she was, at that time, in the last stages of phthisis, those lungs were probably ulcerated, and possibly some irritating matters may have escaped with the expired air, and have been inhaled by the husband.

PRACTICAL CONSIDERATIONS, ARISING FROM THESE CASES.

While we may feel assured that contagion, as held by Morgagni and the Italians, is, at least in this country, a delusion—we may feel, I think, equally assured that we should warn a wife or a sister or near female friend from devoting herself too closely to the attendance upon a consumptive husband, sister or friend. For the sake of the attendant as well as the sick one, sleeping in the same bed, or even in the same room, should be avoided. If, however, this cannot be prevented, then we should try to eliminate all deleterious influences as much as possible. The room should be thoroughly ventilated and cleansed daily. The attendant should eat regularly and pay especial attention to the digestive system. The diet should be nourishing and simple. It would not be amiss for her to take some wine daily. She should walk daily out of doors, and not confine herself to the sick chamber week after week without release. In actual attendance she should beware of inhaling the breath of the invalid. Disinfecting agents might, with advantage, be used in the spittoons. In a word, every good hygienic influence should be brought to bear upon the attendant. At the same time I would have the community understand that, with such care, there is scarcely a trace of danger in any case, save that of a sister, or a wife whose husband is so miserably exacting or thoughtless as to demand that she should sleep with him during his illness. The danger of the health being injured in these latter cases is great, even if the above hygienic rules be strictly adhered to. The best plan is not to allow a sister or a wife ever to take the *sole* charge of the invalid. Whenever it is possible, let a regular hired attendant assume all the harder work, and sleep in the room, if need be, at night, or, still better, in an adjacent room. The wife or sister should be in the room only during the day, and even then with proper and regular intervals of removal to the fresh air. These rules it may often be impossible to carry out; still oftener, they *will* not be. Nevertheless, I believe our cases fully show that they are simply rational and right, and rules that the contagionist and anti-contagionist ought alike to adopt.

PUBLIC HEALTH
IN
AMERICA

An Arno Press Collection

Ackerknecht, Erwin H[einz]. **Malaria In the Upper Mississippi Valley: 1760-1900.** 1945

Bowditch, Henry I[ngersoll]. **Consumption In New England Or, Locality One of Its Chief Causes** and **Is Consumption Contagious, Or Communicated By One Person to Another In Any Manner?** 1862/1864. Two Vols. in One.

Buck, Albert H[enry] (Editor). **A Treatise On Hygiene and Public Health.** 1879. Two Vols.

Boston Medical Commission. **The Sanitary Condition of Boston:** The Report of a Medical Commission. 1875

Budd, William. **Typhoid Fever:** Its Nature, Mode of Spreading, and Prevention. 1931

Chapin, Charles V[alue]. **A Report On State Public Health Work,** Based On a Survey of State Boards of Health: Made Under the Direction of the Council on Health and Public Instruction of the American Medical Association. [1915]

Davis, Michael M[arks], Jr. and Andrew R[obert] Warner. **Dispensaries:** Their Management and Development. 1918

Dublin, Louis I[srael] and Alfred J. Lotka. **The Money Value of a Man.** 1930

Dunglison, Robley. **Human Health.** 1844

Emerson, Haven. **Local Health Units for the Nation.** 1945

Emerson, Haven. **A Monograph On the Epidemic of Poliomyelitis (Infantile Paralysis) In New York City In 1916.** 1917

Fish, Hamilton. **Report of the Select Committee of the Senate of the United States On the Sickness and Mortality On Board Emigrant Ships.** 1854

Frost, Wade Hampton. **The Papers of Wade Hampton Frost, M.D.:** A Contribution to Epidemiological Method. 1941

Gardner, Mary Sewall. **Public Health Nursing.** 1916

Greenwood, Major. **Epidemics and Crowd Diseases:** An Introduction to the Study of Epidemiology. 1935

Greenwood, Major. **Medical Statistics From Graunt to Farr.** 1948

Hartley, Robert M. **An Historical, Scientific and Practical Essay On Milk, As an Article of Human Sustenance:** With a Consideration of the Effects Consequent Upon the Unnatural Methods of Producing It for the Supply of Large Cities. 1842

Hill, Hibbert Winslow. **The New Public Health.** 1916

Knopf, S. Adolphus. **Tuberculosis As a Disease of the Masses & How To Combat It.** 1908

MacNutt, J[oseph] Scott. **A Manual for Health Officers.** 1915

Richards, Ellen H. [Swallow]. **Euthenics:** The Science of Controllable Environment. 1910

Richardson, Joseph G[ibbons]. **Long Life and How To Reach It.** 1886

Rumsey, Henry Wyldbore. **Essays On State Medicine.** 1856

Shryock, Richard Harrison. **National Tuberculosis Association 1904-1954:** A Study of the Voluntary Health Movement In the United States. 1957

Simon, John. **Filth-Diseases and Their Prevention.** 1876

Sternberg, George M[iller]. **Sanitary Lessons of the War and Other Papers.** 1912

Straus, Lina Gutherz. **Disease In Milk:** The Remedy Pasteurization. The Life Work of Nathan Straus. 1917

Wanklyn, J[ames] Alfred and Ernest Theophron Chapman. **Water Analysis:** A Practical Treatise on the Examination of Potable Water. 1884

Whipple, George C. **State Sanitation:** A Review of the Work of the Massachusetts State Board of Health. 1917. Two Vols. in One.

Selections From Public Health Reports and Papers Presented at the Meetings of the American Public Health Association (1873-1883). 1977

Selections From Public Health Reports and Papers Presented at the Meetings of the American Public Health Association (1884-1907). 1977

Animalcular and Cryptogamic Theories On the Origins of Fevers. 1977

The Carrier State. 1977

Clean Water and the Health of the Cities. 1977

The First American Medical Association Reports On Public Hygiene In American Cities. 1977

Selections from the Health-Education Series. 1977

Health In the Southern United States. 1977

Health In the Twentieth Century. 1977

The Health of Women and Children. 1977

Minutes and Proceedings from the First, Second, Third and Fourth National Quarantine and Sanitary Conventions. 1977. Four Vols. in Two.

Selections from the Journal of the Massachusetts Association of Boards of Health (1891-1904). 1977

Sewering the Cities. 1977

Smallpox In Colonial America. 1977

Yellow Fever Studies. 1977